THE
HISTORY OF
MEDICINE
IN 100
FACTS

CAROLINE RANCE

First published 2015

Amberley Publishing
The Hill, Stroud
Gloucestershire, GL5 4EP

www.amberley-books.com

British Library Cataloguing in Publication Data.
A catalogue record for this book is available from the British Library.

ISBN 978 1 4456 5003 6 (paperback)
ISBN 978 1 4456 5004 3 (ebook)

Typeset in 10.5pt on 13.5pt Sabon.
Typesetting and Origination by Amberley Publishing.
Printed in the UK.

THE FACTS

INTRODUCTION

The history of medicine is a vast subject encompassing the whole of humanity in every region of the globe. For millennia, our ancestors have sought to combat disease, relieve pain and postpone the Grim Reaper's inevitable victory, doing so with a fortitude and humour that makes their experiences resonate with us today. The different aspects are all so fascinating, however, that it can be difficult to decide where to start.

The purpose of *The History of Medicine in 100 Facts* is to provide that starting point. The book gives concise introductions to some of the well-known (and not so well-known) episodes from medicine's long history, dispelling a few myths and celebrating a few neglected figures along the way.

1. This Is the Story of Medicine ... Except It Isn't

Every good story has a beginning, a middle and an end. It has a plot, and some characters and lots of conflict. It has coherence, a sense that early events foreshadow those of later chapters and that everything is moving forward towards an outcome that the storyteller has known about all along.

The history of medicine itself has a history, and it's one involving stories. In the late nineteenth and early twentieth centuries, the discipline was led by members of the medical profession, who were often accomplished researchers but also had a habit of polishing the tombstones of the illustrious figures who had represented their profession through the ages. Medical history became a big 'march of progress' story, celebrating all the challenges doctors overcame to get to our current state of supposed medical enlightenment. Important discoveries sprang from the 'eureka!' moments of geniuses, who struggled alone against benighted critics, finally achieving vindication in the acknowledgement of their achievements from a modern perspective.

This view of the history of medicine as a narrative of heroes and villains is so outdated that it's even getting clichéd for historians to criticise it. Medicine never reaches a point at which we've 'made it' – there can be no end to the story until the last human being surrenders to its sentient robot overlords (and even they will no doubt need their aches and pains oiling once in a while).

Patients' own experiences and the role of the huge variety of informal healers now get plenty of attention from historians. Yet heroic stories remain compelling. The figure of the maverick practitioner scorned by reactionaries is still widely popular – for example, when promoting sales of the latest non-evidence-based treatment.

Discoveries are rarely moments of inspiration; they are a collaborative process involving decades, centuries or even millennia of setbacks and breakthroughs, chance observations and targeted investigations. Not only that, but plenty of people have been involved in medicine without having any long-lasting impact at all, but simply by responding to suffering. So this book is not intended to be a 'Top 100 Greatest Medical Advances in the World Ever', nor a '100 Most Heroic Medical Heroes'. Some of the episodes and people included didn't make that much impact on 'progress'; they are here as snapshots of how people approached healing in different contexts at different times.

For reasons elaborated by basic numeracy, a book about 100 things can't cover the billions of events, ideas and people associated with medicine's history – those included are influenced by my own interests and I will inevitably have missed out someone's favourite. I hope any disappointed readers will find it in their hearts to survive. What I have tried to do is introduce some of the key figures and theories in medicine's history alongside some less familiar aspects. The thread that weaves them together is not a narrative of progress but our shared human nature.

2. Prehistoric People Needed Surgery Like a Hole in the Head

An astounding collection of antiquities filled Señora Zentino's palatial home in the Plaza de San Francisco, Cuzco, Peru. She was renowned for her hospitality to travellers and her amusing stories. In 1865, American archaeologist Ephraim George Squier (1821–88) arrived to view the collection – and went away with a skull tucked under his arm.

The skull, from an Inca cemetery at Yucay, dated from around 1400–1530 BCE and had a rectangular hole in its frontal lobe. A piece of bone was missing from the centre of four criss-crossed grooves; it looked like a hash symbol or a noughts and crosses grid. It must have been made deliberately. Squier shared the skull with the New York Academy of Medicine and with French neuroscientist Paul Broca (1824–1880). Broca confirmed that this was not a funeral ritual, but a form of surgery called trepanation, and the patient had lived for two weeks afterwards.

In nineteenth-century hospitals, skull operations were tricky; infection almost always set in. The idea that a supposedly primitive people could have carried out such careful surgery was difficult for some to accept, especially those who considered themselves racially superior to indigenous Americans. Broca, however, was convinced that there had existed 'in Peru, before the European era, a surgery already very advanced.'

Trepanned skulls have been found worldwide, suggesting that the procedure emerged independently in many cultures. The oldest specimens date from around 10,000 BCE in North Africa, and there are also examples from sub-Saharan Africa, North and South America, Europe, China, the Middle East, Russia and Australia.

With so much trepanning going on, it's no surprise to find lots of methods. You could scrape away at the skull with a sharp flint; bore a circle of holes to make a perforated disc; create a round groove or four straight ones (like on the Yucay skull) and pop the middle out. From the time of the ancient Greeks onwards, the surgeon could use cylindrical instruments that rotated to saw out a perfect circle of bone.

Trepanation began before the development of writing, so evidence for its purpose relies on archaeological finds, later descriptions, and its more recent use in indigenous communities. The ancient Greek Hippocratic Corpus (*c.* 400 BCE) mentions trepanning for skull fractures, and in Renaissance Europe it was used to treat epilepsy and mental health problems.

Broca speculated that prehistoric trepanation had a spiritual aspect – had these ancient peoples believed they were allowing demons to escape from the skull? The idea is still popular and plausible, but also risks assuming that the beliefs of ancient cultures conformed to nineteenth-century stereotypes about 'primitives' and 'savages'.

Also possible is that trepanation was a practical therapeutic skill for treating injuries. With head wounds a frequent consequence of conflict or accident, practitioners could have observed the course of infection and realised that dead bone would eventually disintegrate (if the patient didn't die in the meantime). Getting the wound clear of bone fragments might have emerged as a logical step in the encouragement of healing, regardless of any spirits floating around.

3. Where There Are People, There Are Parasites

Since before humans were even humans, we have walked hand in hand with parasites. From head lice to intestinal worms to protozoa, freeloading creatures have entwined themselves into our evolutionary history.

Some were bequeathed to us by non-human ancestors – the threadworm, still the subject of the dreaded letter home from school, cheerfully irritated the bottoms of prehistoric primates. Others got picked up along the way through early humans' food habits. Archaeological evidence – usually in the form of faecal remains (coprolites) – yields a lot of information about parasitic infection, which can even be used to trace our ancestors' migration patterns across the globe.

The earliest known intestinal worms that might be from humans were found in the Grande Grotte of Arcy-sur-Cure, Burgundy, in the 1990s. Coprolites dating from between 24,000 and 30,000 years ago contained the eggs of large roundworms. Other finds show the widespread distribution of infection – 10,000-year-old roundworms have turned up in South Africa and Cyprus, with many more examples appearing across the centuries, often alongside whipworm infection.

Roundworms were less common in the prehistoric Americas, and some researchers have suggested that this is due to medicinal plants such as *Chenopodium*, which was enough to keep them at bay in an environment free from the overcrowding and poor sanitation of later cities. Parasites enter the written record from 1500 BCE, when the ancient Egyptian medical text now known as the Ebers Papyrus included wormwood, pomegranate and castor oil among its anti-worm treatments.

They say that the dog is man's best friend, but the roundworm has stuck with us through thick and thin without so much as a biscuit bone for its faithfulness. Unfortunately, the relationship is not a happy one. These foot-long pinkish-white creatures still infect more than a billion people today, causing intestinal obstruction, malnutrition, haemorrhage due to larval migration in the lungs, and other potentially fatal complications.

Yet perhaps parasites could be put to work for a more positive outcome. In recent decades, scientists have investigated whether worm infection could improve cases of autoimmune disease and allergies. Across the millennia, intestinal worms evolved means of preventing their hosts' immune responses from destroying them. By excreting chemical compounds that tell the immune system to calm down, they give us the side benefit of reducing dramatic reactions to other things – such as peanuts and dust mites. In regions of the world with good sanitation and medical care, the lack of parasitic infection might be enabling people's immune systems to overreact to everyday antigens. Early studies have shown potential for the therapeutic use of parasites such as hookworms, whipworms and blood flukes against allergies and autoimmune diseases including multiple sclerosis, irritable bowel disorder and type I diabetes.

This doesn't mean we should all rush to dodgy clinics in Mexico for a dram of worm eggs (yes, such places have already sprung up on the back of these tentative scientific findings). Globally, intestinal worms are far from being our best buddies and treatment will need to be highly regulated. Under controlled circumstances, however, our squirmy evolutionary companions could be forced to earn their keep.

4. STONE AGE DENTISTS DRILLED OUT DECAY

As anyone who has ever suffered a severe toothache knows, there comes a point when having your entire jaw cut off would feel like a blessed relief. It would also be fatal, which is probably why Stone Age people didn't do it. They did, however, engage in some dental work, and recent studies have shown that it was more sophisticated than previously thought.

In April 2006, a communication published in *Nature* by Alfredo Coppa et al. revealed the earliest known examples of dental intervention. Evidence from a graveyard in Mehrgarh, Pakistan, showed that a farming community living between 7,500 and 9,000 years ago used flint-headed tools to drill holes in molar teeth. Nine individuals – four women, two men and three of undetermined sex – had a total of eleven drilled teeth between them. Smoothing of the hole-margins showed that the teeth had continued to be used for chewing after the procedure, so it must have been done while the people were alive.

The researchers theorised that the holes had been filled with medicinal herbs or a longer-lasting filling, but it was impossible to tell; any such substances had long since rotted away (if they were ever there at all). In 2012, however, studies of a European Neolithic jawbone revealed some exciting new knowledge – a hole in a canine tooth had been filled with beeswax.

This jawbone was found in a cave near Lonche, Slovenia, in 1911 by Giuseppe Müller, an entomologist based in Trieste, Italy. Since then, it had maintained a low profile at Trieste's Natural History Museum. X-ray studies in the 1930s broadly dated it to the Stone Age, but it wasn't until a century after its discovery that new technology could reveal its fascinating dental secrets.

A multidisciplinary research team from institutions in Italy and Australia, led by Federico Bernadini and Claudio Tuniz, established that the jawbone dated from between 6,400 and 6,655 years ago and belonged to a man aged between twenty-four and thirty. His teeth were in pretty bad shape, with areas of exposed dentine. A vertical crack in his canine tooth extended into the inner enamel and dentine as far as the top of the pulp chamber. In other words: ouch! The unfortunate man must have been in such pain that he could hardly eat. No wonder he tried to do something about it.

Synchrotron radiation imaging revealed a substance covering the top of the cavity, and subsequent analyses showed this to be beeswax – not only that, but it dated from the same time as the jawbone so had not got stuck there accidentally in the intervening centuries. Either the man himself or another operator had filled the tooth, probably in an attempt to reduce its sensitivity. The team did not rule out the possibility that the beeswax was added after the man's death as part of a funeral ritual, but their research strongly suggests that the community around Lonche in 4500 BCE knew a thing or two about teeth.

5. COPPER AGE PEOPLE MIGHT (OR MIGHT NOT) HAVE USED TATTOOS FOR HEALING

'I feel sorry for him,' the excursion guide said wistfully. 'But ... c'est la vie.' We were about to go into the South Tyrol Museum of Archaeology at Bolzano, Northern Italy, to say hello to Europe's oldest mummified corpse.

Ötzi the Iceman is a revelation and an enigma. Discovered in 1991 by hikers who thought he was a recently deceased climber, Ötzi – nicknamed for the Ötzal Alps – had lain undisturbed for 5,300 years. He and his possessions were in a remarkable state of preservation that has enabled researchers to piece together his last days. We know he was about forty-five years old – knocking on a bit for a Copper Age chap – and that he had dental disease, intestinal parasites, Lyme disease and degeneration of the lumbar spine.

Just as intriguing is the fact that Ötzi was murdered. He had been engaged in combat before his death, and died from blood loss from an arrow wound. The physiological details are there, but mystery still surrounds the circumstances – what was the killer's motivation? Why was Ötzi up in the mountains, far from home? What went through his mind as he trekked through dangerous conditions, perhaps aware that someone had it in for him?

Such matters for speculation can give us a compelling sense of affiliation with Ötzi's experience; yet he also remains distant, and some aspects of his health status have proved controversial. He has numerous tattoos that could have a medicinal purpose – but conclusive evidence has yet to emerge. Grouped as simple lines or crosses, the tattoos are mostly positioned over joints where Ötzi's diseases would have caused him pain. Researchers initially thought they were a way of introducing plant medications, but it's now known that the tattoos were etched in charcoal, not herbs.

Frank Bahr of the German Academy for Acupuncture and Auriculomedicine was struck by the proximity of the tattoos to traditional acupuncture points. Bahr was part of a team who published articles in *Science* (1998) and the *Lancet* (1999), reporting that nine of the fifteen known tattoo groupings were on or near traditional acupuncture points. Two more were on acupuncture meridians, one was a local point and three were between six and thirteen millimetres from the nearest point.

Based on this one study, it has become widely accepted that Ötzi's tattoos were an early form of acupuncture, pre-dating Chinese acupuncture by around 2,000 years. But is this just a case of 'believing is seeing'? There are a lot of acupuncture points and if you prod yourself in fifteen places you might well hit a few. We don't know for certain what beliefs Ötzi's culture had about tattoos and there remains the possibility that they had a different symbolic or spiritual meaning – or that he just liked them.

In January 2015, a multispectral imaging study by the Institute for Mummies and the Iceman revealed all Ötzi's sixty-one tattoos, including a previously undiscovered group without any obvious health connection. This has set the groundwork for further investigations into their role. They might remain a mystery forever, but let's hope they reveal some secrets about ancient European culture and medicine.

6. Some of the Earliest Known Doctors Were Women

Saqqara is a huge archaeological site about twenty miles south of present-day Cairo. Five millennia ago, it was the necropolis for the ancient Egyptian city of Memphis, and remains home to one of the oldest surviving buildings in the world – the step pyramid of Djoser.

Impressive though the step pyramid is, we need to wander off to another nearby tomb, for that's where we'll find the person we're looking for – Merit Ptah, the first female doctor known by name.

Merit Ptah lived in approximately 2700 BCE and the tomb shows her image with hieroglyphs denoting 'the Chief Physician'. That's pretty much all that's known about her career, but the inscription reveals that it was possible for women to hold high-status medical roles in Ancient Egypt.

Some 200 years later, another doctor, Peseshet, was immortalised on a monument in the tomb of her son, Akhet-Hetep, a high priest. Peseshet held the title 'overseer of female physicians', suggesting that women doctors weren't just occasional one-offs. Peseshet herself was either one of them or a director responsible for their organisation and training, which would happen at the *per-ankh*, or House of Life, an administrative and educational hub attached to many of the temples.

Although the barriers of time and interpretation make it difficult to reconstruct the day-to-day practice of Merit Ptah and Peseshet, it's clear that female doctors were a respected part of society. We shall see later in this book that people in other periods of history didn't always feel the same.

7. ANCIENT EGYPTIAN MEDICAL SPECIALISTS INCLUDED THE 'HERDSMAN OF THE ANUS'

Magic, religion and rational science mingled without contradiction in Ancient Egyptian medicine. A sick person could consult a doctor (called a *swnw*), a magician or a lay priest of one of the goddesses, Sekhmet and Serqet, associated with healing – or all three depending on what felt like the best option at the time. One practitioner might be both priest and doctor, curing via a combination of medicines, incantations and prayers.

Egypt's system of medicine was the first to be set down in writing, but its history remained obscure until hieroglyphs started being decoded in the early nineteenth century. Since then, papyri and depictions in tombs have shown that doctors had an extensive knowledge of disease and a rich pharmacopoiea of herbs, animal products and minerals. Prescriptions were prepared according to precise recipes that could include long lists of ingredients and their measurements, and took many forms including pills, ointments, inhalations and enemas.

One doctor particularly skilled in administering these enemas was Irenakhty, who lived in approximately 2150 BCE. He was doctor to the royal palace and held the position of *neru pehut* – herdsman or guardian of the anus. Other titles listed on his false door (once part of his tomb) were 'doctor of the eyes,' 'doctor of the belly' and 'interpreter of liquids in the *netnetet*'. As yet there's no precise translation for *netnetet* but it is thought to be a sac-like organ and, given the context, probably refers to the bladder.

Irenakhty was not alone in his proctological expertise; his predecessor Khuy was another anal shepherd, who also looked after the top end of the alimentary canal with his skills as a dentist. Dental disease was widespread and a practitioner like Khuy would mainly use pastes packed around the teeth rather than doing anything too invasive.

The Greek historian Herodotus visited Egypt around 440 BCE and remarked on the level of medical specialisation – to him, it appeared that each doctor was responsible for one type of disease. The list of titles for doctors like Irenakhty, however, suggest that there was not such a clear distinction. It's possible that doctors collected extra areas of expertise throughout their career, rather than specialising from a broad base.

Because physicians to the nobility and royalty got fancier burials, they are over-represented among the doctors we know about today. Ordinary *swnw* worked in less exalted positions and were more like general practitioners, dealing with whatever the day threw at them. Renef-seneb, who lived during the Twelfth Dynasty period in the early second millennium BCE, was doctor to the quarry workers at Serabit el-Khadim on the Sinai Peninsula. We can only guess whether or not that was preferable to wrangling with the pharoah's posterior.

8. Papyri Reveal the Earliest Written Surgical Cases

The most important pieces of evidence for ancient Egyptian medical practice are the papyri that came to light during archaeological investigations in the late nineteenth and early twentieth centuries. Twelve papyri, from different sites and dates, survive on medical themes. Although that's not many considering the extent of ancient Egyptian civilisation, they do provide information about the diseases encountered, the substances used in medical treatments and the process of diagnosis and prognosis. Sometimes they also mention now-lost medical texts, suggesting that the ancient Egyptian physician had a substantial body of medical literature at his or her disposal.

The surviving papyri are mostly written in hieratic script, a simplified form of hieroglyphics suitable for use in everyday documents. One of them, the Kahun gynaecological papyrus, found in 1889 at al-Lahun near Luxor, is the oldest known medical text from anywhere in the world. It dates from around 1800 BCE and explains how to treat a variety of ailments specific to women. For example, an aching of the rear, front and calves indicated discharges of the womb and should be treated with a boiled mixture of carob fruit, pellets and cow's milk for four days.

Egyptian physicians did not carry out major surgery and, unlike the ancient Greeks and later societies, there was no separate role of craftsman-surgeon either. They were, however, skilled at treating wounds and orthopaedic trauma.

The Edwin Smith Papyrus, written *c.* 1600 BCE, gives forty-eight case reports of injury. Unlike in other papyri, the text rarely invokes magic or appeals to the gods (there is just one incantation to be used alongside treatment for a fracture of the facial bones). This could be because the type of injury involved left no doubt about what had happened – if you fell off a pyramid or got coshed by an enemy, there was nothing very mystical about it.

The doctor's first step was to examine the patient, palpating the injury and observing its extent. Flesh wounds were sutured, dislocated joints put back, arm fractures realigned with traction and splints, and broken ribs left well alone. The final stage of treatment was often to apply a dressing dipped in oil and honey, keeping the wound moist and acting as a barrier to infection.

Each injury fit into one of three categories: 'an ailment I will treat', 'an ailment I will contend with' (i.e. a difficult case but worth a punt) and 'an ailment not to be treated', where there was little hope of recovery or where doing nothing was just as good as doing something. A severe head wound exposing the brain, for example, was sprinkled with oil and observed until nature took its course either way.

The Edwin Smith Papyrus starts with head wounds and works its way down the body, but only gets as far as the arms and chest when the text abruptly stops mid-sentence. Was the scribe violently dragged from his desk? Did a better-paying job come in with a tight deadline? That remains a mystery, but his hard work is still invaluable to historians 3,600 years later.

9. Prosthetics Helped People Walk (Like an Egyptian)

Ankhefenmut served as priest and sculptor in the temple of the goddess Mut sometime during the period 1069–945 BCE (Egypt's Twenty-first Dynasty). When he died in his early fifties, he was embalmed and wrapped, and placed in an inscribed coffin ready for his bodily resurrection and acceptance by Osiris.

In 1909 a pair of mummies – one of whom was Ankhefenmut – arrived at the Albany Institute for History and Art in New York. He enjoyed a new lease of death until 1989, when a misinterpretation of X-ray investigations suggested he was female. Ankhefenmut was evicted from his coffin and usurped by the other (male) mummy. Fortunately for the researchers, he does not appear to come equipped with a curse.

He is, however, equipped with a false big toe on his right foot. No one has identified how he lost the digit but the replacement is made of ceramic and resin-covered wood and is longer than a natural toe. It's not the first known example of a human-made toe from ancient Egypt, either.

In 1881, the British Museum acquired an artefact from the Reverend Greville Chester (1830–92), a collector with extensive knowledge of Egyptian antiquities. The Greville Chester toe is made from cartonnage – linen fabric set with a binding medium called gesso. It has a tan-coloured coating and was originally fitted with a separate toenail, since lost. The type of linen suggests it dates from before 600 BCE. No information survives about the person who used it but the toe shows signs of wear and evidence of a method for attaching it to the foot. Typical ancient Egyptian sandals would have helped to hold it on and covered the join where it met the foot.

Then in 1998, a survey of tombs in the Valley of the Nobles near present-day Luxor found an even more sophisticated prosthetic toe, which is now in the Egyptian Museum, Cairo. Its owner, a woman aged between fifty and fifty-five, suffered from arteriosclerosis – a hardening of the blood vessels that restricts blood flow and can cause gangrene. The toe might have dropped off naturally or been surgically amputated – either way, it healed and the woman was fitted with a realistic-looking prosthesis with a carved toenail and a dark brown painted coating to match her skin. The main part of the toe attaches by seven leather strings to two wooden plates that articulate with the foot, allowing for movement as the woman walked. It was held on by a broad textile strip and dates from between 1069 and 664 BCE.

Dr Jacky Finch of the University of Manchester carried out a study in 2011, in which volunteers who had lost a toe put replicas of the Greville Chester and Cairo toes into action, showing that these prostheses were designed for practical use.

As for Ankhefenmut, his toe is more likely to have been added after his death to enable him to stride into the next life intact. Thanks to curators at the Albany Institute, he's now back in his rightful coffin and no more mummy-swapping is afoot.

10. Ancient Mesopotamian Medicine Treated Body and Soul

'Why is this happening to me?' the sick person might lament. 'What have I done to deserve this?' Part of the remit of ancient Mesopotamian medicine was to answer these questions – and yes, you had done something to deserve it.

Mesopotamia – not a country but a region made fertile by the rivers Tigris and Euphrates, and covering modern Kuwait, Iraq and northern Syria – was home to many different civilisations during the first three millennia BCE. In parallel with the Egyptians, they developed systems of writing using cuneiform scripts made by pressing a wedge-shaped stylus onto clay tablets. Around 1,000 surviving documents deal with medicine, revealing the presence of a well-organised medical profession.

Or rather, two professions – the *asu* and the *asipu*, who made different but complementary contributions to peoples' health. Both were healers and their activities overlapped, but broadly speaking the *asu* dealt with bodily illness and the *asipu* took care of spiritual wellbeing.

Both practitioners were steeped in a culture that explained disease in terms of retribution – you had done something wrong (often accidentally) and annoyed a specific god, ghost or demon. This entity might actively punish you or, if they were a protective god, they might take the hump and leave you to your own devices.

Using magical information such as omens encountered on the way to the patient's house, the *asipu* made diagnoses, gave prognoses and assisted the sufferer through rituals and incantations.

It all now sounds, well … a bit woo. But within its context it had positive psychological effects for the patient. Anxiety about what they'd done to bring on the sickness was replaced with a sense of clarity and a purposeful way forward. Healing rituals could have improved the patient's state of mind and altered their perception of their symptoms.

The other type of practitioner, the *asu*, used a botanical pharmacopoeia and surgical interventions, though he too could include incantations.

One famous source that illuminates medical practitioners' role is the Code of Hammurabi, a legal document written in Akkadian on a tall stone slab and dating from *c.* 1760 BCE. Nine of its 282 laws mention doctors, showing that their fees were standardised and set on a sliding scale according to social status. An operation to remove a tumour from the eye, for example, cost a freeborn man ten shekels, a freed man five shekels and a slave two shekels (to be paid by the owner). This, however, was only if it turned out well – if the patient died, the doctor risked having his hands cut off (or having to pay for a replacement slave).

Herodotus wrote in the fifth century BCE that the city of Babylon did not have any physicians; instead, the sick sat in the marketplace and were regaled with the advice of random people who had suffered the same thing. No doubt ill people did get just as much 'helpful' advice as their modern counterparts, but the evidence of ancient Mesopotamian cuneiform documents suggests they had an established system of professional assistance to turn to as well.

11. Sight-Saving Surgery Was Possible Six Centuries BCE

Another very old medical text is the *Sushruta Samhita*, written in Sanskrit in India. Its exact date is tentative, as no original version survives and it is only known from later copies, but the current consensus is that it was written in around 600 BCE. Sushruta is thought to have been a physician and teacher working in the North Indian city of Benares (now Varanasi in the state of Uttar Pradesh). His *Samhita* – a compilation of knowledge – gives detailed information on medicine, surgery, pharmacology and patient management.

The *Sushruta Samhita* is a foundation text of the ancient Indian system of medicine called Ayurveda (the knowledge for lengthening the lifespan). Its view of the body is based on the system of the three *doshas* – Vata or Vayu, Pitta and Kapha. Vata is the nerve force that animates the body, pitta is a heating quality that governs the metabolism and kapha is a cooling humidity that relates to moistness in the body such as mucus and phlegm. A derangement of any or all of these doshas leads to disease. An excess of spoiled blood might also imbalance the system, and for these cases, the *Sushruta Samhita* recommended bloodletting.

Perhaps the most remarkable aspect of the *Sushruta Samhita* is its focus on surgery. Sushruta advised his students that, however well-read they were, they wouldn't be competent to treat disease without practical experience. Surgical incisions were to be practised on the skin of fruit, while extracting fruit seeds enabled the student to develop the skill of removing foreign bodies from flesh. They also practised on dead animals and on leather bags filled with water. The students had to perfect their bandaging skills on a life-size mannequin made of stuffed linen before they were let loose on real patients.

Among its many surgical descriptions, the *Sushruta Samhita* documents cataract surgery. The patient had to look at the tip of his nose while the surgeon, holding the eyelids apart with thumb and index finger, used a needle-like instrument to pierce the eyeball from the side. It was then sprinkled with breast milk and the outside of the eye bathed with a herbal medication. The instrument was used to scrape out the clouded lens until the eye 'assumed the glossiness of a resplendent cloudless sun.' After the operation the eye was dressed with clarified butter and a linen bandage.

As well as giving detailed surgical instructions, Sushruta advised on caring for the patient during convalescence. The bandage should be replaced every fourth day and the eye gently bathed with a decoction of botanic drugs. It was important for the patient to avoiding coughing, sneezing, burping or anything else that might cause pressure in the eye. If the operation were a success, the patient would regain some useful vision, albeit unfocused.

With 184 surviving chapters covering 1,120 medical conditions, the *Sushruta Samhita* is a classic of ancient medicine and surgery. Sushruta could not only restore lost eyesight, but lost noses too, and we'll be meeting him again in Fact 46.

12. HIPPOCRATES REJECTED SUPERNATURAL THEORIES OF DISEASE

Lauded as the father of medicine, embodying the ideal of the ethical physician and still influencing the philosophy of modern medicine through his titular oath, Hippocrates must have been quite a guy. Yet, for someone so important, very little information survives about his life. He is thought to have been born on the island of Kos in *c.* 460 BCE and died around eighty-five years later, but even these scant details are 'based on traditional use only'.

What we do have is the Hippocratic Corpus, a collection of more than sixty medical treatises that vary in outlook but share a rejection of the idea that gods caused and cured disease, an acknowledgement of the importance of lifestyle to health, and the concept of the four humours as an explanatory mechanism for the body's wellbeing. They had many authors, who might even have included Hippocrates, and (apart from a few later additions) had been brought together at the great library of Alexandria by 250 BCE.

The Hippocratic tradition framed medicine as both an art and a science. The physician was nature's assistant, supporting the patient's recovery by attending to regimen – the system of diet, exercise, bathing and sleep most appropriate to the individual case. Medicines formed the next line of treatment; surgery was reserved for when there was no other option. The Hippocratic doctors did not usually carry out surgery themselves – surgeons were craftsmen, rather lowlier in social status than the writers of the Corpus.

The physician's identity included his sense of duty to the patient, as exemplified in the Hippocratic Oath, which required its adherents to behave with propriety and confidentiality and to ensure their treatment did not cause harm. (Although the famous phrase 'First do no harm' does not appear in the oath, it reflects the Hippocratic ethos perfectly.) Modern versions of the oath, updated to reflect contemporary medical practice, are still taken by new doctors today, but are not compulsory.

Diagnosis and prognosis were other strengths of the Hippocratic teachings. Listening to patients' own description of their symptoms was important, but so was observing the objective signs of disease on the body – a process doctors had previously neglected. An ability to predict the outcome of an illness no longer relied on purported mystical powers but on observation, knowledge and experience.

To the followers of Hippocrates, disease was a natural phenomenon that had nothing to do with divine punishment, as earlier medical outlooks had assumed. One of the Hippocratic writers was critical, for example, of epilepsy's reputation as a 'sacred disease' caused by a visitation of the gods. This, he said, was an ignorant point of view put about by those who used their religiosity to claim superior knowledge and authority. Under Hippocratic teaching, epilepsy was caused by phlegm building up in the brain and turning it wet and humid. Although this is now known not to be the case, it was a rational explanation within the context of the time and formed an important secular departure from the idea that deities were smiting people with sickness.

13. The Four Humours Began a 2,000-Year Reign over European Medicine

The notion of *humours* underpinned European medical practice from the time of Hippocrates right up to the mid-nineteenth century. The Hippocratic writers called them *chymoi* (juice), referring to the fluids of phlegm, blood, yellow bile and black bile. 'These make up the nature of his body,' wrote the author of *On the Nature of Man* (who was possibly Hippocrates' son-in-law Polybus), 'and through these he feels pain or enjoys health.' Humours were already around as a philosophical concept but *On the Nature of Man* sharpened up the idea into four identifiable components, and the theory was refined by later writers including Galen and Ibn Sina.

Each individual body contained its optimum mixture of these substances, and when they were in balance the person was bright-eyed and bushy-tailed. An excess or depletion of one or more humours, however, caused disease. This theory of health, which had parallels in Indian and Chinese systems of medicine, was a natural philosophy that saw the body as a unified mechanism and departed from the previous tendency to view it as a collection of individual parts.

The number of humours harmonised well with other aspects of nature and life. They fluctuated according to the four seasons. Winter, with its snotty colds, went hand in hand with phlegm; blood surged in the spring when the sap was rising; yellow bile spilled forth in the vomiting bugs of summer, and black bile reflected the decay of autumn. There were four natural elements too – water, air, fire and earth, which corresponded to phlegm, blood, yellow bile and black bile respectively. The humours became associated with four different types of temperament into which people could broadly be classified – phlegmatic, sanguine, choleric and melancholy – and one's age also had an effect on which humour predominated. People between the ages of twenty-five and forty-five, for example, were most under the mastery of black bile; they were prone to quartan fevers, which struck in the autumn.

The physician's job was to restore the balance of the humours by setting out a regimen to counteract the type of disease. Cold, wet, phlegmy illnesses needed warming medicines such as thyme and hyssop, while hot, dry fevers benefited from sloppy food. The idea that everything was related to everything else framed the human body as a microcosm of nature. Humoral theory remained the dominant way of understanding health and sickness for over two thousand years, and many of the drastic treatments of later centuries make more sense when approached from this perspective.

14. Diocles Extracted Barbed Arrows with a Spoon

The Ancient Greek surgeon might have had a lower social status than the physician, but he made up for it with a stomach of steel. Warfare was ruthless, and the battlefield formed a high-pressure arena for surgical developments.

Heavily armoured soldiers called hoplites adopted a phalanx formation in combat, using their shields for defence, but enemy archers could still get in the occasional hit – and a barbed arrowhead in the flesh was bad news. Diocles of Carystus is credited with an invention for removing these missiles without causing even worse damage in the process.

Diocles lived in the fourth century BCE and, although not much of his work survives, fragments of his writings and references by other authors show he was a prolific and thoughtful medical author and a practical physician.

The Dioclean *kyathiskos*, or spoon of Diocles, was a long iron or bronze probe ending in a slim curved scoop with a hole in it. The surgeon would slide the scoop between the arrow and the flesh and manoeuvre it so the arrow's point got caught in the hole. The sides of the scoop, moulded to curve inwards, covered the barbs of the arrowhead, preventing them from ripping the flesh on the way out. By hooking his fingers into two handles at the other end, the operator could pull the projectile out of the body, reducing the chances of infection. Although it's not clear how widely the invention caught on, it appears to have survived for at least 500 years and illustrates how warfare has often required an inventive surgical response.

15. THE OLDEST KNOWN CHINESE MEDICAL BOOK IS STILL IN USE TODAY

Why were people in the first century BCE less healthy than their ancestors? According to an ancient Chinese medical book, it was because they drank too much alcohol, didn't have a balanced diet, neglected their sleep and were preoccupied with instant gratification. *Plus ça change.*

The *Huang Di Nei Jing*, or *Yellow Emperor's Inner Classic*, was compiled in the second and first centuries BCE from a body of knowledge dating back further. Huang Di himself, although usually translated as the 'Yellow Emperor' was not so much a political ruler as a mythological hero akin to a deity. He was said to have lived in the third millennium BCE, and his purported involvement in the *Inner Classic* leant it authority. It is now recognised to be the work of several anonymous authors who wanted to build a comprehensive collection from earlier texts and oral tradition.

The *Huang Di Nei Jing* is divided into two sections, each containing a series of conversations between Huang Di and one of three advisers – principally the royal doctor, Qi Bo. The first section, the *Su wen*, or 'Basic questions', shows Huang Di enquiring about health and human beings' relationship to the universe; keen to learn, he wants to store up the knowledge and pass it on to future generations. The second section, the *Ling shu*, gives practical information about acupuncture, which was beginning to supersede bloodletting in early Han-era China as the cultural emphasis shifted from ideas about obstructed blood to those of an optimum flow of *qi* through the body's channels and meridians.

Qi (pronounced chi) refers to a vital energy or life force present in all things. In the *Huang Di Nei Jing*, the healthy body maintains a balance of *yin-qi* and *yang-qi*. Yin is a quiet, passive force, encompassing feminine qualities and those of cold, moisture, winter and night-time, while yang is sunny, active, masculine and noisy. They complement each other rather than struggle for dominance, but if they become unbalanced, disease moves in.

In the *Su wen*, therefore, the prevention of disharmony is paramount – as the character of Huang Di points out, waiting until a disease arrives before treating it is like digging a well when you are already thirsty, or forging weapons after the battle has started. Through following a simple life, regulating one's activities to the seasons and nourishing the body with good food and sleep, one could maintain the balance and be healthy. It sounds simple, but people evidently weren't managing it 2,000 years ago any more than they are now.

During the first millennium of its existence, the *Huang Di Nei Jing* was not one single book – different writers included different components. The text as it survives today was finished in 762 CE by the author Wang Bing, who spent twelve years arranging it into one coherent whole. In the eleventh century, China's Imperial Editorial Office issued an authoritative version, and this is still a seminal reference work for modern practitioners of Traditional Chinese Medicine.

16. A GENTLEMAN PHYSICIAN INTRODUCED MEDICAL LATIN

For centuries, scholars have debated whether or not the Roman aristocrat Aulus Cornelius Celsus (*c.* 25 BCE – *c.* 50 CE) was actually a doctor. His influential book, *De Medicina* (*On Medicine*), is the only complete surviving section of his encyclopaedia covering subjects as diverse as jurisprudence, the military and agriculture.

De Medicina is the first known medical work in Latin. Celsus' elegant writing style and detailed descriptions make it the foremost historical source for Roman medical practice. Writing at a time when most medical texts were in Greek, Celsus created Latin equivalents of Greek words, many of which became standard medical terms. For example, he translated the Greek *tuphon enteron* (blind gut) as *intestinum caecum*, which has become the *caecum* we all know and love.

Did he really have in-depth personal knowledge of all his topics, or was he repackaging earlier works? None of Celsus' contemporaries describe him as a physician. If his other writings had survived, would we also see him as a farmer, lawyer, soldier and orator? That's a lot to fit in to the day, even for an independently wealthy Roman.

Yet *De Medicina* indicates that Celsus did practise medicine in some form at a time when there was no particular qualification for becoming a doctor. Dedicated individuals could learn medicine through private study, enabling them to treat friends and family without making a career of it. Celsus probably knew what to do when a household member fell ill, but did not need or want to charge strangers for his services.

17. Dioscorides Catalogued the Drugs of the Roman Empire

The Greco-Roman physician Pedanius Dioscorides (c. 40–90 CE), compiled a comprehensive reference work that remained in use in European and Arabic medicine until around 1600 CE. He is often referred to as the 'father of pharmacology' because of the influence of his work on later pharmacopoeias. (NB Lots of figures in the history of medicine get called the 'father' of this or that, sometimes for flimsy reasons.)

Dioscorides' *Perì üles iatrichès*, now known by its Latin title *De Materia Medica* (*On Medicinal Substances*) was not about disease but about drugs. Comprising five books, it catalogued over 800 items, more than three quarters of which derived from plants and the remainder of animal or mineral origin. Most substances could be used in several different ways, so there are around 4,740 therapeutic actions described in the books. Dioscorides arranged his material in an innovative way, grouping the substances by their physiological effects rather than, say, by plant habitat or appearance. He did not, however, elucidate his method of categorisation and some later translators rearranged the work into alphabetical order. From the original Greek, the books were first translated into Latin and Arabic and later into German, French, Italian and English. Exquisite illustrated editions were also produced, for example the *Vienna Dioscurides* manuscript, created in Constantinople c. 512 CE and now housed at the Austrian National Library in Vienna.

Dioscorides came from Anazarbus in Cilicia, Asia Minor, a Greek-speaking province of the Roman Empire. He is traditionally seen as an army medic whose travels during military service gave him the opportunity to gather the native plants of many regions. This might well be true, but the evidence is slender. In his preface to *De Materia Medica*, he does say he travelled widely and lived a 'soldier's life', suggesting some connection with the Roman army, but beyond this there is little biographical information. (He could even mean that he travelled about *like* a soldier in the cause of botany.)

His concise entries give a botanical description of each plant together with information about where it can be found, what effect it has on the body, what to combine it with for different purposes, and what names the plant is known by in different cultures. He occasionally includes magical remedies such as amulets but also displays scepticism about certain traditions; he gives short shrift to the belief that burying powdered ram's horn will cause asparagus to spring up. Where appropriate, Dioscorides also warns about side effects – Greek beans, for example, were a useful ingredient in medicines for bladder stones, scrofulous tumours and breast inflammation, but they caused bad dreams and flatulence.

De Materia Medica is an important source for information about the medicines used in the Roman Empire in the first century CE. It remained a principal textbook until Renaissance herbalists began to record their own observations; even then, the new herbal remedies were evolving from Dioscorides' work rather than overwriting it.

18. Galen Influenced Medicine for a Millennium ...

Hippocrates marked out the path of medicine, but Galen revealed the true way. At least, that is, according to Galen, who could never be accused of having low self-esteem. His confidence paid off, for he became the dominant authority of European and Arabic medicine until the new anatomical discoveries of the Renaissance began to undermine his influence. Even then, his profile remained high as late as the nineteenth century.

Unlike Hippocrates, Galen (*c.* 129 – *c.* 217 CE) left autobiographical detail. He was born into a wealthy Greek family in Pergamon (Bergama in present-day Turkey), and devoted his life to medicine in his teens when the healing god Asclepius visited his father in a dream. After travels in Greece and Alexandria, learning from eminent medical teachers, he became physician to Pergamon's gladiators (a prestigious and gory job). In his early thirties, the ambitious Galen left for the bright lights of Rome, where he became a prominent intellectual and the Emperor's son's personal doctor.

Galen's ethos was Hippocratic – he subscribed to the idea of the four humours, and expanded them to encompass the four temperaments (phlegmatic, sanguine, choleric and melancholic). He, too, emphasised the importance of observing objective clinical signs such as the pulse and urine when making diagnoses.

But whereas the Hippocratics avoided surgery and anatomy (with the result that they did not know much about the body's inner workings), Galen was an expert surgeon and his motivation to carry out dissections bordered on the fanatical. Cutting up human cadavers was forbidden under Roman law, so Galen used monkeys, along with anything else he could get his hands on, including cats and dogs, pigs, goats, snakes, ostriches and at least one elephant. Galen's gruesome vivisections (events full of spurting blood, screaming animals and noisy hecklers) took place before audiences of students, rival doctors and public figures. Ruthless in his infliction of suffering, Galen used such occasions to expose the flaws in other writers' anatomical treatises.

The use of animals sometimes resulted in erroneous assumptions about human anatomy, but also enabled Galen to confirm or reject existing ideas. One of his most famous experiments was on the recurrent laryngeal nerves, providing evidence that the brain controlled the functions of movement and sensation in the rest of the body. Many doctors believed this to be the case but, in the absence of evidence, others followed the competing theory that the heart was the seat of the body's functions.

In Pergamon, Galen was vivisecting a pig when he accidentally cut the laryngeal nerve, making the pig stop squealing even though it was still alive. He was invited to repeat the demonstration in Rome for an audience of intellectuals. This was postponed when the philosopher Alexander Damascenus expressed his scepticism and Galen did an epic flounce. Later, however, the procedure went ahead and Galen replicated his original results. The experiments illustrated the importance of confirming hypotheses through testing.

Galen's career embodied a spirit of enquiry that emphasised original thinking and experimentation, so it was ironic that his writings were to acquire the status of dogma for hundreds of years.

Not everyone, however, accepted his teachings uncritically ...

19. ... But Al-Razi Had Doubts about Him

Abu Bakr Muhammad ibn Zakariya al-Razi had doubts about Galen. So much so, that he wrote a book called *Doubts about Galen*.

That's not to say Al-Razi (854 – *c*. 925 CE) wanted to cut the Greco-Roman anatomist down to size just to be awkward – his own medical education owed a great deal to Galen. But Galen emphasised the importance of comparing one's own observations to the accepted wisdom, and not just blindly following what had gone before. Al-Razi felt that Galen would have welcomed his criticisms and encouraged his independent thinking.

Al-Razi (later referred to in the West as Rhazes) arrived late to a medical career, becoming a doctor in his thirties. He rose to prominence in his home town of Ray (in present-day Tehran Province, Iran), and directed the hospital there, going on to a similar role in Baghdad. This gave him the opportunity to observe large numbers of patients and to carry out treatment trials to see for himself whether standard therapies made any difference. He selected groups of patients with similar conditions and compared their disease outcomes with Galen's descriptions – often he discovered that Galen (who based his observations on only a few patients compared with Al-Razi's thousands) was inaccurate about how diseases progressed.

Al-Razi's freethinking ideals permeated all his works, of which there were many. He wrote at least 200 books and treatises in Arabic and Persian, not just on medicine and chemistry, but on religion (including some robust criticism of the Qu'ran), philosophy, and astronomy too. In one of his most influential works, the *Kitab al-Hawi fi al-Tibb*

(*The Comprehensive Book on Medicine*), he described a trial of bloodletting on patients with suspected meningitis – one group received the treatment and another did not, showing that Al-Razi recognised the importance of a control group. In this instance, the patients who were bled did better, so Al-Razi felt confident in recommending bloodletting for future similar cases. Of course, many variables might have affected the outcome, but it is an interesting early example of the need to test a treatment rather than accepting it unquestioningly.

The theory of the four humours prevailed in medieval Islamic medicine just as it had for the Greeks and Romans, but while Al-Razi adhered to it overall, he also realised that the case for humoralism wasn't watertight. When someone had a hot drink, for example, this didn't unbalance the system by the exact amount of heat in the liquid, but seemed to provoke the body to regulate its own temperature – a contradiction to the humoral idea that the body accepted whatever heat or cold was thrown at it.

Al-Razi's contributions to medicine go far beyond anything we have space for here – among other things, he pioneered hospital psychiatric wards, consolidated earlier Arabic work on the distinction between smallpox and measles and wrote a self-help book for those without access to doctors. A theme that weaves through his work, however, is that of rational thinking and using investigation to confirm or refute even the most entrenched of theories.

20. TRANSLATION RESCUED ANCIENT WORKS FROM OBLIVION

Debate about the works of antiquity was possible because the society Al-Razi inhabited was a hive of cultural and intellectual activity. Later referred to as the Islamic Golden Age, the ninth to eleventh centuries CE saw a focus on the transmission of knowledge throughout the Muslim world, which, at its height, stretched from the Iberian peninsula (Al-Andalus) to as far east as present-day Uzbekistan and Pakistan. The translation of ancient Greek medical texts into Arabic meant physicians like Al-Razi could discuss them, write commentaries on them and build upon them to create original works.

Many people contributed to the 'translation movement', but the most influential in both East and West was Hunayn ibn Ishaq (808–73 CE). He was a Nestorian Christian from Al-Hira, a town about a hundred miles south of the Eastern Caliphate's capital, Baghdad, where Hunayn went to study medicine with an eminent physician. His tutor, however, kicked him out for constantly bugging him with questions (and perhaps for showing the potential to compete with said teacher for court patronage). He then travelled for a while, and returned to Baghdad fluent in Greek.

Hunayn was still in his teens when he began translating the works of Galen into Syriac. Galen was not unknown in the Arab world before this – some Syriac versions of his treatises were already available thanks to the sixth-century physician Sergius of Reshaina – but Hunayn's work expanded the number of texts available and rendered them in Arabic too.

Hunayn has sometimes been associated with the Bayt al-Hikma, or House of Wisdom – the Caliph's library and centre for scholarship in Baghdad, renowned for the translation of Persian texts into Arabic – but the evidence for his involvement there is slim. He did, however, work with his son Ishaq ibn Hunayn, his nephew Hubaysh ibn al-Hasan al-A'sam, and a team of other assistants to produce high-quality translations – together they brought the writings of Galen, Hippocrates, Dioscorides, Plato and Aristotle, as well as other scientific and theological works into circulation.

Hunayn aimed to produce coherent and readable texts, which meant avoiding verbatim translations and instead finding the most accurate version of manuscripts before conveying their meaning in the most appropriate way for their new audience. This could take a lot of legwork – he described travelling around Mesopotamia, Syria, Palestine and Egypt in a futile search for Galen's *De Demonstratione*, only finding half of it in a scruffy manuscript at Damascus. On that occasion he was unlucky, but his dedication undoubtedly saved many works that would otherwise have been lost.

Perhaps with his own glorious exit from medical education in mind, he created a practical revision text called *Questions on Medicine*, presenting Galenic and Alexandrian medical concepts in a handy Arabic Q & A format. The book was perfect for helping students remember information, and *Questions on Medicine* became an official text for medical exams. It was so useful, in fact, that centuries after Hunayn's death it was central to the revival of Galen's ideas in the medieval Christian West.

21. Anglo-Saxon Medicine Involved Leeches (Who Didn't Suck Blood)

Meanwhile, in the Anglo-Saxon kingdoms of what was to become England, the medical practitioner was called a *læce* – a leech. This probably has a different origin from the word for a pond-dwelling worm (whom we will meet properly in Fact 65) but the human leech was just as central to healing. Although active at the same period of history as the prolific Arabic translators and polymaths, the Anglo-Saxon leech left behind far less evidence about his (or her?) theories and everyday practice.

Few individual Anglo-Saxon doctors can be identified. The best-known early English medical text, *The Leechbook of Bald* (*c.* 950 CE) mentions two, Oxa and Dun, who taught medical recipes to the book's compiler. The book was put together by a scribe named Cild on the instructions of Bald, so it's reasonable to suspect that Bald, a literate man, practised as a leech too – or at least had a sincere interest in medicine. Each formula or procedure is called a leechdom, and references to other unnamed leeches suggest there was an active exchange of medical learning, even if it wasn't a formal system of education.

Bald's *Leechbook*, plus other surviving works called *Leechbook III* and the *Lacnunga*, show that Anglo-Saxon leeches mixed complex recipes involving botanical and animal products, used Christian rituals, and drew on their pagan heritage to sing charms. (Christianity took hold in England during the course of the seventh century, but did not wipe out cultural memory). As the saying goes, a problem shared is a problem halved, and the litanies and charms probably helped the patient articulate their fears and feel more hopeful about the outcome. It is not useful to try and divide Anglo-Saxon medicine into our modern 'rational' and 'superstitious' distinctions; they were part of the same thing.

Theories about the cause of disease drew both from classical literature and from the pre-Christian Anglo-Saxon culture. Practitioners were familiar with the four humours and the hot, cold, dry and moist elements that accompanied them, but this theory was less prominent than it became in the later Middle Ages. While humoral theory attributed disease to an imbalance within the body, the Anglo-Saxons recognised that it could strike from the outside too, as in the case of 'flying venom', for which there were many treatments.

This phenomenon was a particular problem at Lammastide at the beginning of August, when 'venomous things fly and much injure men'. In the middle of the summer, infectious diseases were at their height and stores of cereal crops were at their lowest before the new harvest, making people vulnerable to disease. Bald's *Leechbook* recommends avoiding bloodletting and medicines around this time, so as not to weaken the body, and to stay indoors during the middle of the day when the air is most impure. Flying venom bears some similarities to the idea of miasma (see Fact 42), and if the 'venomous things' were insects rather than malevolent spirits or abstract concepts, it could implicate the malarial mosquitoes on the rampage at that time of year.

22. Ibn Sina Brought Together All the Medical Knowledge of His Time

Back in the Arab world, Galen's teachings continued to dominate medicine, but the increasing availability of ancient texts made it clear that he and the natural philosopher Aristotle (384–22 BCE) contradicted each other a lot. Abu Ali al-Husayn Ibn Abd Allah Ibn Sina (980–1037 CE) addressed this problem while bringing together up-to-date knowledge from different medical traditions in one comprehensive text.

Ibn Sina (later referred to in Europe by the Latinised name of Avicenna) was born near Bukhara, now in Uzbekistan but at that time under Samanid Persian rule. He studied medicine privately and became a doctor at the age of just seventeen. In spite of getting caught up in political machinations and having to make himself scarce on a regular basis, Ibn Sina wrote a lot – 240 works survive and he produced many others that are since lost. The work that sealed his reputation as a medical authority was *Al-Qanun fi' al-'Tibb* (*The Canon of Medicine*).

Natural philosophy – the study of nature and the universe – shared fields of interest with medicine. Anatomy, for example, revealed information about the creatures of the natural world and about disease. Galen's study of anatomy, although flawed, had revealed information unavailable to Aristotle, and running through Ibn Sina's work is a commitment to reconciling Aristotle's philosophy with the medical knowledge of Galen. On points where they clashed, Ibn Sina tended to follow Aristotle – for example, in the idea that the heart was the body's centre of control.

The *Canon* explained Galenic medicine, but it didn't just rehash Galen's own ideas; it presented them in the context of tenth-century knowledge, and drew on Indian, Arabic and probably Chinese contributions to elucidate the ancient concepts.

Ibn Sina organised the *Canon* into five books. The first explained humoral theory and gave an overview of the causes of disease, and how to prevent and treat it through diet and lifestyle. When regimen failed to keep the body in good health, however, it was necessary to use medicines, and Book Two catalogued around 800 plant, mineral and animal substances used in pharmacology. Book Three dealt with diseases affecting specific parts of the body, while Book Four covered injuries and systemic conditions such as fevers. Finally, the last book gave around 650 formulae for compound medicines, using the ingredients detailed in Book Two. This elegant organisation contributed to the books' usefulness in medical study.

As well as being a prolific writer, eminent philosopher and esteemed physician, Ibn Sina was an incorrigible party person, and his excesses caught up with him in his late fifties. He died at Hamadan, Iran, in 1037.

The *Canon* was translated into Latin in the thirteenth century by Gerard de Sabloneta (also referred to as Gerard of Cremona, and not to be confused with the other Gerard of Cremona, who translated scientific texts in the twelfth century. Unless, of course, it was one bloke who had some kind of secret potion for longevity.) Gerard's translation of the *Canon* entered the university medical curriculum of medieval Christian Europe and remained influential well into the early modern period.

23. MAIMONIDES COULD HELP YOU THWART ASSASSINS

Moshe ben Maimon, born *c.* 1135 in Cordoba, Andalusia, is one of the most influential Jewish philosophers ever to have lived. His renown rests chiefly on his code of religious law and ethics, the *Mishneh Torah*, and on the *Guide for the Perplexed*, reconciling religious and philosophical concepts.

But Maimonides (the Latinised form of his name by which he is now known) was also a physician, whose prolific writing took place around a hectic schedule of patient consultations. As well as his philosophical works, he wrote ten medical books – including a practical toxicology guide.

Maimonides' childhood in Cordoba came to a turbulent end when the city was captured by the Almohad Caliphate, and after many years of travelling, his family ended up in Fustat – now part of Old Cairo. Maimonides, who had studied medicine throughout his unsettled youth, gained the patronage of al-Qadi al-Fadil, advisor to the Sultan, and became the court physician. Not only that, but he was appointed to the prestigious judicial role of Head of the Jews in Egypt. He was one busy person.

A typical day was exhausting. Up early to go to the palace, he would deal with the royal household's ailments and not get away until afternoon. Once home in Fustat, he would grab his only meal of the day and get started on the hordes of patients waiting for him. Sometimes these consultations went on after nightfall and, in a letter to one of his students, Maimonides described having to lie down with fatigue while listening to his patients and making prescriptions. Somehow, Maimonides still found time to write.

His *Treatise on Poisons and their Antidotes* was commissioned by al-Fadil as a public information project in 1198. The bites and stings of snakes and scorpions posed a very real threat in Egypt, and the *Treatise* was designed as a first aid handbook so people could improve the victim's chance of survival while waiting for a physician. It described, for example, the use of a tourniquet and a method of sucking out the venom.

Poison, as well as venom, was a danger – especially to those in high-profile roles abounding with enemies. Maimonides gave advice on remaining alert to the use of strongly flavoured and colourful foods, which were perfect for would-be assassins to disguise their nefarious activities.

Maimonides claimed not to be contributing anything new to toxicology, but to be presenting existing information in a clearer way. His treatise, however, does show the importance of thinking critically about received wisdom. It was common practice, for example, to give unleavened bread to victims of scorpion bites or stings – Maimonides pointed out that there was no evidence for the benefits of this.

The Treatise on Poisons and their Antidotes is not Maimonides' most important work in terms of its influence on posterity, but it was important if you were an ordinary medieval Egyptian who had just been bitten by a venomous snake. In spite of – or because of – his erudition, he was able to make medical information accessible to those who needed it.

24. Ibn Al-Nafis Discovered the Pulmonary Circulation

One day in the public baths of thirteenth-century Cairo, a bather suddenly got out, went to the changing room and asked for pens, ink and paper. He sat down, wrote an entire treatise about the pulse, then went back and carried on with his bath. This anecdote from a fourteenth-century biography, whether true or not, exemplifies the astonishing productivity of Ala-al-din abu Al-Hassan Ali ibn Abi-Hazm al-Qarshi al-Dimashqi, known to his friends as Ibn al-Nafis (1213–88). Ibn al-Nafis was a critical thinker who argued against the accepted Galenic ideas about blood's movement in the body.

Born near Damascus, Ibn al-Nafis studied medicine there before moving to Egypt in 1236. He wrote several original books, including eighty volumes of a planned 300-volume encyclopaedia of medicine, but his particular genius lay in interpreting and commenting on existing works. He wrote commentaries on various parts of the Hippocratic Corpus, Hunayn ibn Ishaq's *Questions on Medicine*, and Ibn Sina's *Canon of Medicine* (among others). Another biographical anecdote describes him writing 'like a down-pouring torrent', discarding each blunt pen and grabbing a new one rather than waste time cutting them. He extracted the anatomical sections from Ibn Sina's *Canon* and brought them together in his *Commentary on the Anatomy of the Canon of Ibn Sina*, criticising their Galen-inspired portrayal of the heart and blood.

Although erroneous, Galen's teachings were an important starting point in the understanding of circulation. Galen believed blood originated in the liver and flowed to the right ventricle of the heart, where a proportion of it would cross through invisible pores in the muscle wall to the left ventricle. There, it mixed with air from the lungs and became 'vital spirit' or *pneuma*, which flowed to the organs via the arteries. The veins, meanwhile, carried the rest of the blood through the body to nourish it. It didn't make a return journey – it was consumed by the tissues and renewed by fresh blood from the liver.

Ibn al-Nafis was adamant that no pores, visible or invisible, connected the two ventricles. He recognised that: 'The blood from the right chamber must flow through the *vena arteriosa* (pulmonary artery) to the lungs, spread through its substances, be mingled there with air, pass through the *arteria venosa* (pulmonary vein) to reach the left chamber of the heart and there form the vital spirit.' He did share Galen and Ibn Sina's belief in this vital spirit necessary for the organs to function.

Ibn al-Nafis wrote that religious law and his personal beliefs did not permit him to carry out dissections, but his in-depth knowledge of the heart's construction suggests that he must have seen the real thing at some point.

European doctors were oblivious to Ibn al-Nafis' work and Galen remained the dominant influence on the continent, but in 1547 some of Ibn al-Nafis's writings were translated into Latin by Andrea Alpago of Belluno. During the next century, further developments enhanced understanding of the blood's circulation, culminating in William Harvey's experimental demonstration of the systemic circulation in 1628.

25. The *Trotula* Gynaecological Texts Were Not Written by Trotula

Salerno in Italy was the undisputed centre of medieval Western European medical education. The prestige of its school, the Schola Medica Salernitana, attracted students from far and wide, and treatises published by the faculty disseminated the most up-to-date medical thinking across the continent. By the twelfth century Salerno's reputation was so exalted that it became known as the 'city of Hippocrates'.

From this vibrant medical milieu emerged an influential text – the *Trotula,* which covered obstetrics and gynaecology and was widely circulated in Europe in the medieval period. The title 'Trotula' became understood as the name of the work's author, thought to be a female practitioner whose insider knowledge of women's health added to the authority of her writings.

But who was this Trotula? Was she really a woman? Did she even exist at all? Over the centuries, the enigmatic figure of Trotula accumulated biographical baggage for which there was little evidence. According to some accounts, she was part of the noble di Ruggiero family, was married to a physician and had two sons. She was also feted as a professor at Salerno medical school – this notion emerged in the late seventeenth century with the work of Salernitan historian Antonio Mazza, who invented it for reasons of his own. With the city of Padua announcing a female PhD in 1678, perhaps Mazza wanted the world to believe that his hometown got there first.

Previous writers had tried to erase the author Trotula altogether. In 1566, a new edition of her works was attributed to a male writer called Eros Juliae, whose role became that of an ancient author justifying male involvement in gynaecology.

It was not until the late twentieth century that historian John F. Benton's analysis of the *Trotula* revealed that it was made up of three texts, all by different writers. They comprise: the *Book on the Conditions of Women* (*Liber de sinthomatibus mulierum*), *Treatments for Women* (*De curis mulierum*), and *Women's Cosmetics* (*De ornatu mulierum*). *Trotula* was the name of this ensemble, not of the author.

De curis mulierum, however, can be attributed to a female writer or compiler named Trota or Trocta. She also produced a general medical work, *Practica secundum Trotam*, which deals with gynaecological conditions and those – including snakebite and insanity – that might affect male or female patients. The most recent research, led by historian Monica H. Green, suggests that Trota was real, she was female and she practised medicine in twelfth-century Salerno. There is no evidence, however, that she taught at the medical school or even had an academic background, and the biographical details of her family and nobility are fictional.

26. Monks Began to See Clearly

The invention of spectacles did not involve a lone genius going 'Behold! I have invented spectacles!' and proceeding to be ignored by everyone and/or burnt at the stake. Like most scientific developments, it was a process, involving many contributions.

In medieval Europe, the need for magnification was most obvious in monasteries, where hours of reading and transcribing took their toll. 'Reading stones' – clear polished glass with one surface flat and the other convex – were developed by Andalusian polymath Abbas ibn Firnas (810–87) in the ninth century and were soon adopted by Catholic monks. The study of optics was well established in both the Islamic world and Europe, and the influence of such writers as Ibn al-Haytham (c. 965 – c. 1040) and Roger Bacon (c. 1214 – c. 1292) set the groundwork for the practical application of corrective lenses.

During the last quarter of the thirteenth century, Italian persons unknown tried fixing two lenses together. Dominican friar Giordano da Rivalto (1260–1311) said in his 1306 Lent sermon that eyeglasses had been introduced within the past twenty years – the ability to make them was 'one of the best as well as the most useful of arts that the world possesses'. Another Dominican, Alessandro da Spina (d. 1313), was credited in his obituary with learning how to make glasses and making them widely available after their original unnamed inventor tried to keep them secret.

The earliest styles comprised two sections resembling magnifying glasses, with a rivet holding the ends of the handles together. These were held up to the face or balanced on the nose – a precarious position that did not respond well to sudden movements. It wasn't until around 1728 that London optician Edward Scarlett introduced side-arms – or at least was the first to advertise them. His beautifully lithographed trade cards show a pair of specs with arms ending in spiral finials that lay flat against the sides of the head; these would later develop into hooks over the ears.

A 1664 book by Ferdinando Leopoldo del Migliore (1628–96) claimed the invention of spectacles for his home city of Florence, attributing it to one Salvato d'Armati who supposedly came up with the idea in 1284. Del Migliore's claims were debunked in the early twentieth century owing to the inauthenticity of his attempts at medieval language.

In 1953, two complete pairs of spectacles, plus several fragments, were found under the floorboards of the nuns' choir in Wienhausen Abbey, Lower Saxony, Germany. Dating from around 1330, they are the oldest known examples of the invention that has become so essential to millions of people's lives.

27. THERIAC CURED EVERYTHING

At the turn of the eighteenth century, one could visit apothecary Richard Stoughton at the Unicorn in Southwark and spend 3s 6d on a pot of Venice treacle. The pots were guaranteed to have been transported unopened from Italy and to contain a product made from the best quality ingredients. It was not, however, the sticky sugary stuff we would now associate with the word 'treacle', but a panacea with roots in the first century BCE.

Being a king in ancient times was exhaustingly dangerous. Someone was always plotting to bump you off for their own gain; even your mum couldn't be trusted. So, according to legend, Mithradates VI of Pontus (a region on the shores of the Black Sea in modern Turkey) attempted to become resistant to poisons and venoms by administering doses of gradually increasing potency. He was also reputed to have conducted toxicological experiments on condemned prisoners, culminating in the creation of *mithridate* or *mithridatum* – a medicine that combined all known antidotes in one potent formula. It didn't work against Roman armies, however, and when Mithradates was defeated by the military leader Pompey in 63 BCE, the recipe arrived in Rome. Emperor Nero's physician Andromachus developed it into a sixty-four-ingredient composition called *galene* ('tranquillity'), which also became known as *theriac*. Initially an antidote to poison, it became a prized (and expensive) cure-all. Giving the recipe in verse, Andromachus revealed that its principal ingredient was viper's flesh. Along with opium, this remained a component of true theriac for centuries to come. Most of the other ingredients were botanical, with a few mineral and animal substances.

Scepticism about such concoctions started early. Pliny

the Elder (23–79 CE), whose encyclopaedia of *Natural History* included medicine, thought the complex formula 'a showy parade of the art, and a colossal boast of science.' A hundred years later, however, Galen was more enthusiastic, and his influence helped to cement theriac's popularity.

Via the Silk Road, theriac became important to Arabic and Chinese medicine as well as to the Europeans. By the twelfth century CE, Venice was a leading exporter and, in England, the substance became known as Venice treacle (a corruption of 'theriacal'). It was a prominent line of defence when the Great Plague hit London in 1665.

But theriac's fortunes would eventually wane. In 1745, British doctor William Heberden wrote a sceptical essay, *Antitheriaka*. His view was that Mithradates had not been that much of a pharmacologist but that after his defeat, some enterprising Romans cashed in on his reputation by inventing a complicated recipe and claiming it had been found among the king's papers. Heberden condemned its inefficacy and the potentially dangerous drug interactions within the formula. After this debunking, theriac was removed from the London Pharmacopoeia but remained in some continental European pharmacopoeias until the late nineteenth century. Informal use of theriacs persisted longer – in 1915, a British newspaper columnist named 'Whist' referred to their popularity among the 'ignorant peasants yonder'.

28. East and West Met at Monte Cassino

The lively intellectual milieu in which medieval Arabic medicine thrived was separated from Europe by barriers of language and politics. While Al-Razi, Ibn Sina and other Persian and Arab writers were adding their own developments to the ancient Greco-Roman traditions, European medicine ticked along in a less illustrious manner. Hippocrates and Galen took a back seat until the mid-eleventh century, when the transmission of knowledge started in earnest between the Islamic and Christian worlds.

That's not to say everyone in Europe sat around going 'duhhhh' for a millennium; medical wisdom continued to pass from one generation of doctors to the next. But when a North African merchant named Constantine visited Italy in the middle of the eleventh century, he found that, although physicians had practical competence, medical textbooks of the sort used in his homeland were severely lacking. Constantine's efforts to rectify this situation ignited a period of translation and scholarship that enabled the emerging universities to develop up-to-date medical curricula. The medical school of Salerno, established in the ninth century and already respected for the quality of its graduates, led the trend.

The exact span of Constantine's life is unconfirmed but he was born in about 1020 CE and died before the end of the century. In Europe, he became known as Constantine the African (this might make him sound like the solitary inhabitant of a whole continent, but it refers to Ifriqiya, the medieval name for a region of North Africa encompassing present-day Tunisia). His early biographers differ in the details of his life and probably incorporated apocryphal elements, but they portray him as a Saracen (i.e. a Muslim) from Carthage. He transported his own collection of Arabic medical texts to Italy in the 1060s or 70s, losing a portion of them in a shipwreck along the way.

Constantine is thought to have converted to Christianity shortly afterwards (although there's a possibility that he was a Christian all along as there were minority Christian communities in Ifriqiya). He became a Benedictine monk at the abbey of Montecassino, about sixty-five miles north of Naples, and it was there that he worked on translating his collection into Latin.

Constantine's translations weren't word-for-word – he reinterpreted and rearranged the texts for a Latin-speaking audience, keeping their Arabic origin at a low profile for diplomatic reasons. Among the most influential of his works was the *Pantegni*, based on the Persian physician al-Majusi's *The Complete Book of the Medical Art* (ironically, Constantine's version remained incomplete as part of his Arabic copy was at the bottom of the Mediterranean.) As well as numerous other works, he adapted the treatises of the Jewish philosopher and doctor Isaac Judaeus, some Galenic and Hippocratic texts, and Al-Razi's *Comprehensive Book of Medicine*.

As someone who had learnt Latin later in life, Constantine had a fairly rough and ready style, and more elegant translations began to appear in the twelfth century. He had, however, led to a resurgence in the exchange of information that would see the ancient classical authors returning to the centre of medical education.

29. A Little Book Taught the Art of Medicine

One of the works attributed to Constantine the African was a medical text called the *Isagoge* (meaning 'introduction'), and it was to become the lynchpin of European medical study for four hundred years. The *Isagoge* got top billing in an anthology of foundational works aimed at helping students grasp the concepts of medicine. This anthology became known first as the *Ars Medicinae* and later as the *Articella*, or *Little Book of the Art*.

Constantine (or one of his contemporary translators) adapted the *Isagoge* from Hunayn ibn Ishaq's *Questions on Medicine*. Hunayn's Arabic version was in a useful question and answer format, whereas the new Latin translation used a straight narrative arrangement, divided into concise sections on such topics as fevers, swellings and the ages of life.

In Salerno in the early twelfth century, the *Isagoge* was bound together with four other works – Hippocrates' *Aphorisms* and *Prognostics*, Theophilus Protospatharius' *On Urines* and Philaretus' *On Pulses*. Although the latter two texts had a practical side to them, the anthology was no instruction manual – it was about the theory and philosophy of medicine and what it meant to be a doctor. The compilation became a handy reference guide for those embarking on a medical career. In the mid-twelfth century Galen's *Art of Medicine* joined the crew and the *Articella* became popular with academics across Western Europe. Over the centuries it was added to and rearranged, but remained the nucleus of university medical education until the middle of the sixteenth century.

30. Urine for a Treat with Medieval Doctors

While it seems pretty sensible to include general medical works in the *Articella*, what could be the significance of Theophilus Protospatharius' *On Urines?* Nothing against urine, of course, but it's a very specific subject to take up one of just five spaces in an introductory textbook.

Theophilus probably wrote *On Urines* in the Byzantine East in the seventh century CE (though it's not known exactly when he lived). He used classical sources such as Galen to bring together a handbook of uroscopy – the practice of diagnosing disease (or confirming good health) by assessing the urine. Hippocrates and Galen had used urine inspection as one part of a more comprehensive medical examination, and it had an important role in Arabic medicine too. In medieval Europe, however, uroscopy really took off, becoming central to what it meant to be a physician. The university-educated doctor needed to perfect the art, or he wouldn't stand a chance of building up a successful practice.

Like later diagnostic tools such as the stethoscope and the X-ray, uroscopy sought to reveal the inner mysteries of the human body. The physician used a clear, bulbous flask called a *matula*, shaped so as not to distort the view of the liquid within. He looked at the colour, the consistency, and the sediment, referring if necessary to a urine chart showing the spectrum of hues. There were numerous combinations of these characteristics, and each permutation indicated a different disease.

Interpreting the urine became a complex job requiring masses of knowledge and skill. To the average patient, a bottle of piss just looked like a bottle of piss, so the physician's ability to glean the body's secrets from it made for an impressive performance. Patients loved it – perhaps it was the perceived objectivity of the practice, or the convenience of being able to send a messenger off with a urine sample while you got on with being ill in peace.

As uroscopy increasingly became the One True Way to diagnose disease, its reputation got shakier – at least among the doctors who had to do it. Less conscientious practitioners enjoyed equal success by 'cold reading' the patient, or just making up any old thing, so there was plenty of competition. Qualified physicians found themselves under pressure to keep diagnosing by urine; if they didn't, they appeared unskilled, and patients would take their pisspots and purses elsewhere. Vigilance against jokers was also essential – anonymous samples of cow urine, wine, etc., were an occupational hazard and could result in extreme embarrassment for the physician and hilarity for the community.

Gradually, uroscopy fell from favour, and polemics such as Thomas Brian's *The Pisse-Prophet, or Certain Pisse-pot Lectures* (1637), assisted its demise. Although some practitioners continued to promote their urine-analysing skills right up to the nineteenth century, the contents of the chamber pot went back to being part of a wider process of assessing signs and symptoms – with the patient actually there.

31. Women Practised Medicine in Spite of Exclusion

As Europe's universities became the gatekeepers to the medical profession, the person holding up the urine-filled *matula* was extremely likely to be male. Women (apart from in a few exceptional cases) were excluded from academia and could not gain a medical degree, regardless of their abilities.

Women did, however, continue to play a central role in treating the sick, as they had always done. Often, this was in an informal capacity such as providing care for neighbours, but women sometimes gained recognition from the authorities. In some Italian regions female healers – especially those who were the daughters or wives of doctors – were granted official licences to practise either as a specialist in one type of disease or on a more general basis. In 1309, for example, Lauretta of Piedmont gained a license to practise several surgical techniques, including lithotomy – a gruesome but survivable operation to remove bladder stones by making an incision in the perineum.

One case from fourteenth-century France, however, shows the challenges facing women practitioners. Jacqueline or Jacoba Felicie (born *c.* 1290), an Italian living in Paris, practised as a physician up to the year 1322 (and perhaps beyond). She defies the modern stereotypes of the historical female healer – she wasn't an elderly 'wise woman' (though they made an important contribution too), she wasn't a midwife, she didn't focus on diseases specific to women, and no one accused her of witchcraft.

We know about Felicie because she clashed with the head honchos of the medical establishment. In 1322, the

Faculty of Medicine of Paris prosecuted her and five other unlicensed practitioners (two men and three women) for practising medicine illegally. The records of Felicie's trial show how she carried out her work, revealing that she was a skilled practitioner whose good reputation spread through the community by word of mouth.

The charges against Felicie were that she visited the sick and used diagnostic techniques such as urine inspection, pulse taking and palpation. She then allegedly made an agreement to cure them and discussed fees. She prescribed medicines and visited the patient regularly, continuing to examine them to see how they were progressing. In other words, she did what a male doctor would do, but apparently with greater success. Her patients reported having consulted qualified doctors first, or spent time in hospital to no avail, only to be cured by Felicie.

To do all this officially, Felicie needed a licence granted by the chancellor of the church and the medical faculty. Yet she couldn't get a licence because women could not go to university to gain the required qualifications. She was fined sixty livres and excommunicated from the church. Although technically the authorities' clampdown affected male unlicensed practitioners too, the 'Catch-22' situation about licensing and universities specifically excluded women from practice. It's not known whether Felicie continued to assist sick people, but if she did, she would have had to use her skills on the quiet.

32. The Great Pestilence Revealed Ugly Truths about Human Nature

When the bubo arrived, you were a goner. You were lining up the bucket on the penalty spot; the worms held their cutlery and drooled.

The bubo, a swelling of the lymph nodes in the groin or armpit, was confirmation that your fever, headaches, chills and muscle pains were in fact bubonic plague – and your last three days on earth were going to be agony.

The Great Mortality or Pestilence (later referred to as the Black Death) arrived in Europe in 1347 from what people generally referred to as 'the East' – now thought to be the steppes of Central Asia. The bubonic form is transmitted by rodent fleas; pneumonic plague can be passed from person to person by infectious droplets in the breath, and septicaemic plague occurs when the bacteria enter the bloodstream. It is likely that the Black Death epidemic encompassed all these forms.

The Decameron by Giovanni Boccaccio (1313–75), written shortly after the plague swept through Florence, is one of the most significant eyewitness accounts of the devastation. The bulk of it is a series of entertaining stories narrated by a party of young noblemen and women who have fled the plague. The introduction, however, gives the backdrop to their situation – the scenes of terror and destruction that consumed Florence like an inferno when the pestilence arrived in 1348.

Medical treatment was futile. Doctors, folk healers and entrepreneurs alike offered remedies, but nothing worked. The municipal infrastructure was efficient at first – officials ordered the clearing of filth from the streets and the isolation of suspected cases. Citizens held prayer events and processions, appealing to God to spare them. He didn't.

Some chose to isolate themselves indoors and live a temperate lifestyle, ignoring bad news from outside. Others adopted an 'eat, drink and be merry' philosophy, going on pub crawls, larking about in dead people's abandoned houses and getting as much pleasure as possible out of life while it lasted. A third option involved some attempt at normality, going about one's business and carrying flowers or spices to cover up the stench of rotten flesh. Finally, many upped and fled, going to the countryside in an attempt to outrun the disease (only to find scenes of unharvested fields, abandoned animals and dying peasants).

Perhaps the most fascinating part of Boccaccio's account, however, is the erosion of community and humanity. It was everyone for themselves. Neighbours who would have helped each other in ordinary times of sickness stayed away. People who abandoned their relatives ended up suffering a lonely death of their own. According to Boccaccio, parents even departed in fear from their dying children.

Is Boccaccio's account reliable? After all, he was (heaven forbid!) a fiction writer rather than a 'proper' historian. But one of fiction's roles is to get to the essential truths about human nature. His insights into the fragmentation of society, the breakdown of relationships, the uneasy confluence of terror and last-ditch merriment make it easy to picture the same fundamental responses occurring again in some future epidemic.

33. An Alarming Disease Broke Out in England … and Then Disappeared

Plague wasn't the only disease that struck with terror. The sickness that affected England five times between 1485 and 1551 was, according to French ambassador Cardinal Jean du Bellay, 'the easiest in the world to die of'. The English sweat, or *sudor anglicus*, could be fatal within hours of the first symptoms. If you made it through a whole day, the prognosis was favourable, but during its first outbreak, 15,000 people died.

John Caius (1510–73), a doctor who witnessed the 1551 outbreak, described the symptoms. Pains in the back, shoulders, limbs and head were accompanied by hot flushes and 'grief in the liver and the nigh stomach'. Delirium and palpitations set in; the patient would be exhausted but unable to sleep. Then there was the profuse sweating that gave the disease its name. Caius saw the sweat as the body's attempt to expel poisons. He recommended that as soon as symptoms started, you should get into bed without even stopping to undress, and wait it out.

Outbreaks occurred in the summers of 1485, 1508, 1517, 1528 and 1551. The 1528 epidemic – in which Anne Boleyn suffered and recovered – was the only one to spread outside England's borders, affecting northern continental Europe too. After 1551, it never returned, although a milder strain appeared in France in 1718.

John Caius associated it with gluttonous lifestyles; later hypotheses (mostly now discounted) have included typhus, influenza, insect-borne arboviruses, ergotism and anthrax. Recent studies lean towards a hantavirus, acquired through contact with infected rodent urine. The severity of the English disease, its sudden disappearance and the difficulty of identifying it have made it an enduring mystery.

34. Queen Isabella Sent Ambulances to War

The need to remove casualties from battlefields was nothing new in 1484. The Romans had whisked injured soldiers away in chariots; a hammock-like set-up between two horses brought fallen Normans to safety.

It is during the expulsion of the Moors from the Iberian peninsula, however, that the first true ambulances are supposed to have been deployed, and Isabella I of Castile (1451–1504) is credited with commissioning them. She did indeed supply *ambulancias* for her troops, but these were mobile field hospitals rather than patient-transport vehicles.

Isabella's marriage to Ferdinand II of Aragon united the northern kingdoms of Iberia and in 1482 they launched military campaigns against the Emirate of Granada, the region's last remaining Muslim state. Ferdinand and Isabella's historiographer-royal relates that at the Battle of Álora in 1484, Isabella funded six large tents supplied with medical equipment and staffed by physicians, surgeons and attendants. Similarly, four hospital tents served the wounded of the 1489 siege of Baza.

An oration by Pedro Bosca after the siege of Malaga in 1487 referred to medical supply wagons following the army. But although his phrase 'quadragenti ferme currus' was translated in the nineteenth century as 'about four hundred ambulances', it is not clear that they were used for transporting casualties. The injured soldiers, however, must have got to the field hospitals somehow, and it's plausible that the wagons doubled up for this purpose.

Isabella's compassion did not extend to the Jews and Muslims persecuted under her reign. Her contribution to military medicine is somewhat overshadowed by her and Ferdinand's establishment of the Spanish Inquisition in 1480.

35. Mercury Was the Top Treatment for Syphilis for over 400 Years

7 April 1579: a twenty-six-year-old man is brought to a surgeon's door in a state of agony. A large nodular swelling distorts his scalp; others rise from his limbs and chest. The roof of his mouth appears eaten away, so ulcerated that he can't drink without the liquid flooding from his nostrils. His shin bones are rotting beneath him and every joint in his body aches so constantly that he has not slept for days. The man, described in William Clowes' *A Brief and Necessarie Treatise* (1585), has the great pox – syphilis.

Although it's now recognised as a systemic bacterial disease, the dramatic symptoms on the surface of the body brought the pox within the remit of the early modern surgeon – who treated external disorders – rather than the physician. Crusty scabs in the hair, ulcers, reddish-brown scales on the palms, decayed finger joints and disintegration of the nose cartilage ... it was all highly visible. When the disease emerged in Europe in the late fifteenth century, the obvious starting point in the search for a cure was the established treatment for leprosy and skin diseases – mercury.

Mercury could be applied as an ointment to the limbs, taken as pills, or used in suffumigation, which involved surrounding the patient with mercuric smoke. The treatment's logic lay in its ability to induce ptyalism – the excessive production of saliva, which would release the 'venereal venom' from the body. To achieve this state, the patient must endure the unpleasant process of what was effectively poisoning.

This salivation treatment often appeared to work because syphilis naturally goes into latent stages before returning with a vengeance months or years later. Yet surgeons became concerned about the tortures their patients were under, and explored the potential of other treatments.

Some surgeons, such as Daniel Turner (1667–1741), preferred a mercury compound called calomel to crude mercury – the latter had the unpleasant habit of going right through the patient's digestive system and reappearing at inopportune moments. Patients might 'find it in their breeches, or on the Ground, if they mist it in the close-stool'.

Early sixteenth-century sufferers enjoyed a vogue for guaiacum, a wood that came from the Americas (where the disease itself was thought to come from) and didn't have the painful side effects of salivation. Patients starting guaiacum treatment after having mercury probably did start to feel better because they weren't being poisoned any more, but practitioners soon began to doubt it was doing any good.

Sarsaparilla, a herbal medicine, was another reputed anti-syphilitic. In 1830, William Lawrence, surgeon at Barts, described it being used in conjunction with mercury treatments, so it was difficult to tell whether it was having any effect. Although opium, sassafras and cinchona bark also had their supporters, mercury remained the first line of attack against syphilis until the early twentieth century. Salvarsan, introduced in 1910, was the first truly effective treatment, and was used until it was superseded by penicillin in the 1940s.

36. The Dose Made the Poison

The German-Swiss physician and alchemist Theophrastus von Hohenheim (1493–1541), now remembered as Paracelsus, was an irascible, troublemaking odd bod born under a wandering star … in a good way. He challenged the medical dogma of his day and applied the principles of alchemy to medicine.

As a youth, he worked for the powerful Fugger family's mining empire, and also learnt from his father, a physician. He then studied (or at least claimed to have done so) at several universities, but the unquestioning acceptance of centuries-old medical texts was not for him; he set out on a quest for knowledge that took him through all parts of Europe (so he said, although there's not much evidence for exactly what he was up to during this period of his life).

Paracelsus rejected the concept of the four humours. Rather than trying to achieve harmony within the individual, he saw the body as a microcosm of Nature's macrocosm. Disease came from external poisons, not from humoral imbalances. The protoscience of alchemy traditionally sought the philosopher's stone – that elusive substance that would turn base metals into gold, but Paracelsus widened the remit of alchemy to find *arcana* – the specific chemical remedies that existed somewhere in Nature for each disease.

Although most drugs were plant-based, minerals weren't unknown in medicine – mercury, as the previous chapter relates, was used for syphilis. Paracelsus, however, went further in applying chemistry to medicine. His use of arsenic, bismuth, antimony, lead, iron and zinc led to criticism from Galenic physicians, who condemned his prescriptions as 'poison, corrosive, and an extraction of all that is evil and poisonous in nature'.

Paracelsus' response has led to him being dubbed 'the father of toxicology'. This is a bit over the top considering people had been studying poisons for centuries (and on a more general note, there's no need for every subject to be the offspring of a sole discoverer), but Paracelsus' theories of toxicity are interesting and insightful. They appeared in the third of his *Seven Defensiones,* a polemic written in 1538 but not published until after his death.

'All things are poison,' Paracelsus wrote, 'and nothing is without poison: the Dose alone makes a thing not poison. For example, every food and every drink, if taken beyond its Dose, is poison: the result proves it.' This was later distilled by others into the catchier phrase 'the dose makes the poison.' The message remains pertinent in these days of scaremongering about the vague 'toxins' that assail us.

In 1527, Paracelsus gained a teaching position at the University of Basel in Switzerland, where he soon annoyed everyone. Within a year, he was out on his ear, and with his medical writings getting banned in various European cities, he adopted the pseudonym Theophrastus Paracelsus for publications concerning astrology. He was back to shifting from place to place, making new enemies and picking up followers. He died in Salzburg in 1541, not having reformed medicine to the extent he intended, but leaving a legacy of chemical medicine that would persist long after Galenic philosophies had fallen by the wayside.

37. China's Materia Medica Contained Nearly 1,900 Drugs

Life is short, and it saves a young person a lot of time and energy to embark on the career they really want rather than the one their parents expect. Li Shizhen (1518–93) spent his teens studying for China's Imperial examinations; his father hoped this would lead him into a prestigious government role. Li's father was a doctor and in Ming Dynasty China even a well-educated and accomplished physician did not enjoy much status; he wanted Li to go up in the world. Fortunately for medicine, Li wasn't cut out for the bureaucratic life – he failed the exams three times and his father eventually agreed to train him as a doctor. Li Shizhen went on to devote much of his life to compiling a giant encyclopaedic work of pharmacology that remained the standard materia medica in Chinese medicine until the mid twentieth century.

The *Bencao Gangmu*, or *Compendium of Materia Medica*, was a monumental fifty-three-volume work completed in 1578. For the past three decades, Li had studied all the available medical works – some 800 books – assessing the accuracy of their information and correcting outdated ideas. His scholarship, however, was not confined to the written word; he also travelled around China learning from informal healers, farmers, herb gardeners and anyone else with knowledge to offer about the remedies used regionally to tackle illness. By doing this, he was able to include in the *Bencao Gangmu* 374 substances that had never before appeared in a pharmacopoeia. Ultimately, he described almost 1,900 drugs, with 11,000 prescription combinations for their use. More than half were of plant origin but there were also animal and mineral drugs, including many derived from the human body. His 'yellow soup', for example, used human faeces as a remedy against diarrhoea, anticipating the faecal microbiota transplants that are now recognised as effective against *Clostridium difficile* infection.

Li did not immediately publish the work – with the help of his sons and grandsons, he took it through two revisions during the 1580s. After Li's death in 1593, his son presented it to the Wanli Emperor, but this reclusive ruler did not do much about it and the first edition was a privately printed one that appeared in 1596. Only in the next century did the magnitude of the work become appreciated and from the 1640s onwards it was widely reissued and translated into many languages.

In spite of Li Shizhen's focus on medicine, he neglected his own health during his decades of toil. In 1580, a scholar whom he approached to help with revising the book described him as 'emaciated' – as though he had been eaten away by a life's work that received little recognition until he was long gone.

38. A 'TREE OF LIFE' CURED SCURVY

February 1536: In a makeshift fort on the banks of the St Lawrence River near the Iroquoian town of Stadacona (now Quebec City), twenty-two-year-old Philip Rougement lay dead. Three ships hung motionless in the river's ice and their crews – 112 men – were in danger of sharing Rougement's fate. Many already showed the symptoms: swollen legs, purplish spots on the skin and, as *Brief Récit et Succincte Narration de la Navigation Faicte es Ysles de Canada* (1545) put it: 'their mouth became stincking, their gummes so rotten, that all the flesh did fall off, even to the rootes of the teeth, which did also almost all fall out.'

When the expedition leader, Jacques Cartier (1491–1557), ordered Rougement's body to be opened, he found the man's heart 'white, but rotten, and more than a quart of red water about it.' Cartier was none the wiser about how to save his crews.

Scurvy wasn't a new disease, but as European explorers struck out to distant lands from the end of the fifteenth century, it made its presence felt. Caused by prolonged deficiency of ascorbic acid (vitamin C), scurvy afflicted sailors who spent months lacking fresh food.

This was Cartier's second voyage to the place he was to call Canada and although he had initially received a warm welcome from the Stadaconan Iroquoians, the French newcomers' presence was causing tension. During his first voyage in 1534, Cartier had kidnapped two brothers, Dom Agaya and Taignoagny, taking them back to France as proof that he had discovered new territory. Now they were home, the men and their community had every reason not to trust Cartier – an attitude he interpreted as 'treachery'.

Paranoid that any local gathering – even for innocuous celebrations – was a plot against him, Cartier did not let on that his men were sick. When he bumped into Dom Agaya and noticed that his former prisoner was in good health after a period of similar illness, he pretended he had an ailing servant and asked for advice about a cure.

Dom Agaya showed him how to make a decoction of a tree called *annedda* and, although the Frenchmen wondered if it was a trick to poison them, some gave it a go and were cured within days. After that, there was such a rush for the medicine that 'they were ready to kill one another', and used up a whole large tree. The present-day identity of *annedda* is not certain but there are several candidates including eastern white cedar and white spruce.

Cartier repaid Dom Agaya by kidnapping him again along with his father, brother and seven other people, and taking them back to St Malo. By the time Cartier returned to Canada in 1541, all but one of the prisoners were dead. The scurvy cure did not gain widespread recognition and the disease continued to claim the lives of sailors for another 250 years.

39. AMBROISE PARÉ TURNED HIS BACK ON BOILING OIL

Getting shot by a hackbut – the precursor of the musket – wasn't something Hippocrates and Galen had to worry about. So as the military use of firearms spread in the fifteenth and sixteenth centuries, surgeons had to adapt old methods to the treatment of a new kind of injury. Influential in this aspect of military medicine was the Italian surgeon Giovanni de Vigo (1450–1525), whose *A Compendious Practice of the Art of Surgery* (1514) included a chapter on gunshot wounds. His methods spawned a famous episode in the history of medicine, in which French surgeon Ambroise Paré (1510–90) is credited with revolutionising surgery.

The details come direct from Paré himself – in his life story, *The Apology and Treatise of Ambroise Paré* (1585), he describes how he initially followed de Vigo's advice to cauterise gunshot wounds with boiling elder oil to eliminate the poisons thought to be in gunpowder. When Paré ran out of oil, he substituted a dressing of oil of roses, turpentine and egg yolks. The next morning, he found that those treated with the dressing were doing better than those whose wounds had been cauterised. Inadvertently, Paré had created two treatment groups whose outcomes he could compare. 'See,' he wrote, 'how I learned to treat gunshot wounds; not by books.'

The incident went down in the history of medicine as a 'Eureka moment' that shifted surgery from butchery to enlightenment. As with many iconic stories, however, there was more to it. Paré had the rose, turpentine and egg mixture handy because it was already an established part of gunshot wound treatment, as recommended by the very Giovanni de Vigo whose methods he was rejecting.

De Vigo's treatment was more detailed than the usual story suggests. He gave three options for bullet wounds – cauterisation with a heated metal instrument, the application of boiling oil of elder, or *unguentum egypticum*, an ointment containing alum, verdigris, vinegar and honey. If cauterising, the surgeon should then anoint the wound with 'a digestyve of terebentine made with oyle of roses, and ye yolk of egges' (English translation by Bartholomew Traheron, 1543). The method included aftercare of the wound, with herbal plasters to assuage pain and protect the site. Paré rightly skipped the most dangerous and painful part of this process, but also maintained the continuity of attempting to prevent infection and make the patient comfortable.

In Turin, Paré sought out an unnamed surgeon famous for his success with gunshot wounds. The surgeon eventually revealed his secret recipe for an ointment made from newborn puppies, earthworms, turpentine and oil of lilies. While not the same as Paré's, it was similar enough to make Paré happy that his accidental discovery was as good as the methods of his more illustrious colleague. In other words, at least one other surgeon was already treating bullet wounds with a topical medicine.

What Paré did differently was to communicate his knowledge and encourage others to ditch cauterisation as well. He wrote a treatise on gunshot wounds in French, not Latin, making it accessible to the average barber-surgeon and thereby promoting the dissemination of surgical knowledge.

40. Mummy Knew Best

If you need a medicinal mineral and can't get hold of any, the obvious solution is to use a human corpse instead. Mumia – or powdered Egyptian mummy – gained an excellent reputation in sixteenth-century Europe for its powers against a spectrum of ailments including bruising and blood loss. No self-respecting apothecary would be without a supply. For Ambroise Paré and several of his contemporaries, however, the popularity of mumia was exasperating and repulsive.

Mumia emerged from some imaginative translations of medieval Arabic texts, followed by a chain of substitutions of the 'next best thing' that ended up departing altogether from the original thing.

Ancient Roman and Greek physicians considered the slightly rude-sounding pissasphalt – a semi-liquid bitumen – to be of medicinal importance. It occurred naturally in the Dead Sea region and at Apollonia (in modern-day Albania), but a particularly prized source was a mountain in Darábjerd, Persia, where the local word 'mumiya' referred to its waxy texture. The medieval physicians Al-Razi, Ibn Sina and Ibn Serapion the Younger all mentioned a bituminous 'mumia', and it was from European interpretations of their writings that corpses began to get involved.

Gerard de Sabloneta, who translated Al-Razi into Latin in the thirteenth century, saw mumia as 'the substance found in the land where bodies are buried with aloes by which the liquid of the dead, mixed with aloes, is transformed and it is similar to marine pitch.'

Liquid of the Dead might be a great band name but it also inspired a shift towards a new concept of mumia – an aromatic substance that exuded from ancient Egyptian corpses and resembled pissasphalt. Indeed, there was a common belief that the Egyptians had used bitumen during embalming and that the bodies were therefore an alternative source. Those local to the sepulchres quickly saw a business opportunity. Before long, not just the exudate but the body itself was being sold as mumia. By the early sixteenth century, mumia was also derived from recently deceased persons who had been dried out by desert storms.

These corpses still didn't meet the European demand, so some merchants began embalming any dead bodies they could get hold of. In the second half of the sixteenth century, European writers began to protest against the use of mumia; debate arose about what the substance really was.

Ambroise Paré was among those who denounced it – mostly on the grounds that it didn't work. Another problem for Paré was that you never knew what you were getting; the mumia could comprise 'the mangied and putride particles of the carcasses of the basest people of Egypt,' or a French criminal hot off the scaffold. Another writer, Leonhart Fuchs (1501–66), described mummy-using doctors as 'stupid' and cursed pharmacies as 'the very offices of hangmen and shops of vultures.'

Over the course of the seventeenth century, mumia fell out of favour, although it remained available to some extent into the twentieth century. Its long history was part of a wider tendency of society to look to the body itself as medicine – a tendency echoed today in transplants and transfusions.

41. Vesalius Revolutionised the Study of Anatomy

The modern graduate might find it a little vexing that, in 1537, twenty-two-year-old Andries van Wesel walked straight from his medical degree into a lectureship at the University of Padua. Van Wesel (1514–64), who Latinised his Flemish name to Andreas Vesalius, had already exhibited a talent for dissection and within a couple of years his reputation as an anatomist and teacher soared.

Anatomy was a big thing in sixteenth-century Italy. Since the rise of the medieval universities as centres for medical education, professors had carried out human dissections in front of eager audiences of students.* Cadavers could be hard to come by, and students might only get to observe one or two dissections, but they also had access to anatomical textbooks – principally *Anathomia corporis humani* by Mondino de Luzzi (c. 1270–1326).

Vesalius' work grew from this receptive milieu, but it marked a turning point. Although anatomy offered room for experimentation and discovery, it still broadly adhered to the teachings of Galen, who had used animals to inform his theories about the human body. Galen didn't make this explicit, so his works appeared to be describing human anatomy. Vesalius became increasingly aware that Galen's descriptions did not match the actual cadavers in front of him. When in 1539 he gained permission to dissect executed criminals, this supply of material helped him to confirm his suspicions. Through demonstrations comparing human and monkey skeletons, he spread the word that Galen had not accurately depicted the human body.

In 1543, Vesalius published *De Humani Corporis Fabrica* (*On the Fabric of the Human Body*), an anatomical textbook based on observation of real-life (or rather real-death) cadavers. The *Fabrica* was no pamphlet for the average bod to flick through on the privy; it was lengthy, Latin and literary – an expensive work of art aimed at the intellectual elite. The clarity of illustration and the physical beauty of the production made it an artistic as well as a scientific masterpiece. It was both acclaimed and criticised, the objections ranging from the accusation that Vesalius had misinterpreted Galen's Greek to the idea that the human body had changed since Galen's time.

The *Fabrica*'s emphasis on observation rather than acceptance of dogma did have its problems. Most students still lacked access to enough dissection material, and practical experience needed to be accompanied with teaching about what all these parts of the body did. Vesalius, however, led the study of anatomy in a direction that prioritised investigation. When later anatomists corrected parts of the *Fabrica*, they were putting its open-minded ethos into practice.

* Some later historians interpreted the 1299 Papal Bull *Of detestable cruelty* as a prohibition on dissection because it forbade the funerary practice of boiling the flesh from bones. As early as 1904, however, the American popular historian James J. Walsh debunked this, arguing that the Bull had never been intended as, or interpreted as, an anti-dissection move. The centre of anatomical study, the University of Bologna, was under Papal control – but the myth of religious persecution continuing into Vesalius' time has proved difficult to bury. While the Catholic Church was hardly a basket of cuddly bunnies, anatomists weren't in its firing line.

42. Miasma Theory Attributed Disease to Poisonous Air

If you were a well-to-do Roman considering building a new villa, location was important – not for proximity to an outstanding school, but to ensure you were well away from marshes and the poisonous breath of the creatures therein. Marcus Vitruvius Pollio (*c.* 70–15 BCE) warned that breezes could bring in the mist from swampy areas, ruining the health of your family. Vitruvius (as he's usually known) wasn't a medic – he was an architect – but he was going by a theory of disease that remained dominant for centuries.

Miasma theory held that poisonous or corrupt air caused illness. Such air rose from decaying animal or vegetable matter or from marshy waters, and it could be carried on the wind to an unsuspecting community in an otherwise healthy place. It explained outbreaks of disease; when lots of people fell ill at once, it made sense that they were all subject to the same damaging vapours.

The concept appeared in the Hippocratic writing *Airs, Waters, Places*, which connected disease with environmental conditions such as stagnant water. The idea paralleled that of ancient Indian and Chinese cultures – in China, the poisonous vapours of *zhangqi* pervaded the humid mountainous areas of the south, causing malaria and dysentery. (Malaria also means 'bad air' and was linked to the idea of miasma, especially as it was prevalent in areas of standing water where mosquitoes breed.)

Yet, even in times of epidemic, not everyone fell ill. Why was this? Galen explained it in terms of individual susceptibility – someone with an imbalance of the four humours became more vulnerable to miasma's baleful influence.

During the time of the Great Mortality (now known as the Black Death) in the fourteenth century, tracts advising the public on avoiding and treating the plague used terms such as 'pestilential air' to describe the cause. Fragrances from nosegays or incense would impede the air's putrefaction. The notion led to some sensible public health measures – in 1388, the Statute of Cambridge made it illegal in the cities, boroughs and towns of England to cast dung, offal, entrails and other ordure into water sources because it was making the air 'greatly corrupt and infect'.

In nineteenth-century Europe, miasma theory held its own against the idea of contagion from person to person. Although they were topics for debate, the theories weren't always mutually exclusive – it depended on the disease. Since its emergence in Europe in the fifteenth century, for example, syphilis had been recognised as the consequence of 'lewd behaviour', and the communicability of smallpox was fundamental to the practice of inoculation (see Fact 53). It was therefore possible to attribute some diseases to contagion and some – such as typhus, typhoid and cholera – to miasma. By the end of the nineteenth century, miasmatic vapours had been superseded by germ theory, which held that microscopic pathogens multiplied in the body. But as we shall see, that didn't come from nowhere – like most discoveries, it was a long process spanning centuries and involving the contributions of many people.

43. SEEDS COULD BE THE CULPRIT TOO

If you or I had coined the word 'syphilis' we might be tempted to sit back for the rest of our lives and congratulate ourselves that our work on this planet was done.

By contrast, the Veronese physician Girolamo Fracastoro (c. 1476–1553), who did coin the word syphilis in his 1530 poem *Syphilis, or the French Disease*, went on to other achievements. In 1546, he wrote *On Contagion, Contagious Diseases and their Cure*, setting out a theory about how disease got from one person to another. His ideas both rivalled and supported the concept of miasma.

'Contagion' didn't spring into Fracastoro's brain from nowhere; the possibility of disease moving from person to person was already out there. Common sense suggested it might not be a good idea to cuddle people with horrible illnesses.

What Fracastoro added was a mechanism for how disease transfer happened. He suggested that 'seeds' of disease passed between people by direct touch, by contact with inanimate things (fomites) that a sick person had used, or through the air.

Although contagion differed from miasma and made for some debate, there was no pitched battle between miasmatists and contagionists. Fracastoro's ideas allowed for the possibility of seeds moving through the air, which fitted well with the notion of bad vapours.

Fracastoro didn't imply that the seeds were living organisms, and it would be inappropriate to describe him as 'ahead of his time' as a proponent of germ theory (like all other ideas, Fracastoro's were part of the time in which he had them). He did, however, form part of the rich intellectual background from which germ theory could later emerge.

44. IDEAS ABOUT CIRCULATION CONTINUED TO CIRCULATE

Because discovery is a process rather than a lightbulb moment, there can be a lot of emotive debate about who was the 'real' discoverer. In the case of William Harvey (1578–1657), who demonstrated the systemic circulation of the blood in 1628, the existence of several precursors might prompt cries of 'Harvey wasn't the first! Ibn al-Nafis was! And so were the ancient Chinese! And Serveto! And Colombo!'

So, who are all these people and what did they say about circulation? We met Ibn al-Nafis in Fact 24; he described the pulmonary transit of blood. The concept of circulation is also prominent in the *Huang Di Nei Jing* (see Fact 15) but there is little evidence that the authors mean a physiological movement of blood through the cardiovascular system – it's a circulation of *qi* through its own channels.

Miguel Serveto (1511–53) was a Spanish doctor and theologian whose criticism of the doctrine of the Trinity excited the outrage of both Catholics and Protestants. In his 1553 work, *Christianismi Restitutio*, Serveto described how vital spirit got from one side of the heart to the other without passing through the septum. This, however, was a theological book, not a scientific one, and his enemies were more concerned with its religious heresies than its biology stuff. The Inquisition tried to get him but he jumped out of the Catholic frying pan into the Calvinist fire and was burnt at the stake in Geneva. With no dissemination of the book, the idea of pulmonary circulation went back into hiding.

Contemporary with Serveto was Matteo Realdo Colombo (*c.* 1515–59), anatomist at the University of

Padua. He probably did not have access to the rare unburnt copies of Serveto's book, though it's within the realms of possibility that he and Serveto knew of each other. It's plain, however, that if something exists, more than one person can find it. Colombo rediscovered the pulmonary circulation and this time the knowledge remained ... in circulation.

Such developments fostered a fertile intellectual climate for the study of anatomy; the presence of valves in the veins also became known during this period. In 1628, Harvey published *Exercitatio Anatomica de Motu Cordis et Sanguinis in Animalibus,* describing the experiments he had been engaged in since at least 1616. Like Galen, on whose work he aimed to expand, he carried out multiple vivisections of animals. He examined the heart in life and near-death, and used ligatures on the blood vessels to establish the direction of flow. Unlike Galen, however, he concluded that the heart pushed blood in a complete circuit round the whole body – and he could prove it experimentally.

The thought of having to say goodbye to a 1,400-year-old system of medicine took some getting used to and Harvey did face opposition. His work, however, was widely accepted before the end of his life. A few years after his death, Marcello Malpighi's expertise with microscopes revealed the existence of capillaries. There was still more to discover, and always will be.

45. The First Condoms Were Worn after the Event

Gabriele Falloppio (1523–1562), of tube fame, taught anatomy at Padua from 1551 until his death from tuberculosis at the age of thirty-nine. A contemporary of Vesalius, he amicably corrected and added to aspects of the *Fabrica*, and made valuable original contributions to anatomical knowledge of the head and reproductive organs.

In this chapter, however, we're concerned with a claim often made on his behalf – that he invented the condom, or was at least the first to describe one in print.

Falloppio was concerned with the prevention as well as treatment of the 'French disease' or great pox – the venereal infection that endangered the unsuspecting gentleman whenever his penis inadvertently fell into the vagina of an irresistible but tainted prostitute. Falloppio's pox treatise *De Morbo Gallico*, published posthumously in 1563, was compiled from his lectures for his anatomy students, and the advice on preventing infection was for use in their personal lives as much as for sharing with their future patients.

Falloppio recommended careful washing of the penis after sex – a practice already known to the more savvy among prostitutes' clientele – and then using a linen covering to marinate the organ in preventive medication.

The linen only covered the glans of the penis and had no function as a barrier between the healthy man and the 'unclean' woman (a gendered dynamic that appears frequently in early modern literature of the pox). The medication was the important part. Falloppio recommended an ointment containing shavings of guaiacum and precipitated mercury (both standard treatments for venereal disease), wine, flakes of copper, red coral, burnt ivory and burnt deer's horn. When soaked in this mixture, the linen cover was ready for use and could be conveniently carried. It was more discreet than whipping out a pot of anti-pox unguent and offending the woman with one's suspicions that she was horribly diseased.

Falloppio's condoms, which were not called condoms, were not used like condoms, and were not actually condoms, have nevertheless gained pride of place as a 'first' in condom history. Condom use prior to Falloppio's time is plausible but unconfirmed; purported depictions in 15,000-year-old cave paintings and in ancient Egyptian art are open to interpretation.

The earliest physical evidence of condoms comes from a latrine at Dudley Castle in the West Midlands, where fragments of ten seventeenth-century johnnies made from animal membrane were sifted from the waste in 1985. It was possible to date the fragments accurately to between 1642 and 1647, when the castle's defences were demolished and the latrine sealed. It's uncertain whether their owners used them primarily for disease prevention or for their contraceptive effect, but one user appears to have been very careful indeed – five of the condoms were layered inside each other, giving quintuple protection.

46. Plastic Surgeons Offered New Noses for Old

Although the term 'plastic surgery' sounds modern, the desire to reconstruct missing parts of the human body goes back to ancient times. The loss of a nose – whether the result of punishment for transgression, unluckiness in sword-fighting, or syphilis – has historically led surgeons to try to restore the patient's features and their dignity.

Gaspare Tagliacozzi (1545-1599), professor of anatomy at Bologna, is a big name in reconstructive surgery. His illustrated 1597 book, *De Curtorum Chirurgia per Insitionem,* described how to recreate a missing nose. He didn't claim to have invented the procedure but he aimed to describe it scientifically and educate other surgeons about it.

Tagliacozzi's operation involved making parallel incisions in the skin of the upper arm and drawing a linen dressing underneath it. After about fourteen days, he cut the flap at one end; another fourteen days allowed the flap to mature and he then engrafted it to the patient's nasal cavity, using a system of bandages to keep the arm and face together. After another two weeks or so, he separated the arm from the nose (much to the patient's relief) and shaped the graft accordingly.

By Tagliacozzi's time, nasal reconstruction had been practised in Italy for about 150 years. It was, however, kept secret by the families who developed it. The first reports of Italian rhinoplasty involve Gustavo Branca of Sicily who, in the early fifteenth century, used a flap of skin from the face. His son Antonio developed an arm-to-face technique that became known as 'the Italian method' and was expanded upon by the Vianeo family in the early 1600s. Neither the Brancas nor the Vianeos published any writings about their methods – that would have been bad for business.

It's not known how the elder Branca learnt to create noses, but a similar practice dated back to at least 600 BCE. The ancient Indian surgeon Sushruta (see Fact 11), used a plant-leaf template to dissect a flap of skin from the patient's cheek, leaving it attached by a strip called a pedicle. Twisting it so the wound surface remained downwards, Sushruta would suture it into the place of the missing nose and affix small reed tubes to serve the purpose of nostrils.

Within his lifetime, Tagliacozzi's methods became famous and his students replicated the procedure, but after his death in 1599, new noses fell into obscurity. It was not until the late eighteenth century that European surgeons realised they were still being created in India.

A letter to the *Gentleman's Magazine* in 1794 told of an army bullock-driver called Cowasjee, who was captured by the sultan and punished as a traitor by having his nose and one hand severed. An unnamed Mahratta surgeon skilfully created a new nose from the skin of Cowasjee's forehead.

Joseph Constantine Carpue (1764–1846) of the Duke of York Hospital, Chelsea, drew upon the reports from India to carry out nasal reconstructions in 1814, after practising on cadavers. The procedure became known as 'Carpue's operation'; his work revived interest in rhinoplasty and helped European surgeons catch up with their Indian counterparts.

47. A Quechua Medicine Tackled Malaria

The Roman Empire had been and gone, but the swamps and their creatures remained. At the beginning of the seventeenth century, malaria was still rife in Rome, and there was no cure.

Malaria is caused by blood-borne protozoa of the genus *Plasmodium*, which travel from one human host to another in the innards of a female *Anopheles* mosquito. *Plasmodium falciparum* is the most deadly of the species infecting humans. Early symptoms can be unspecific fever, chills, headaches and nausea, but can progress to life-threatening anaemia and respiratory distress.

In early modern Europe, the disease's parasitic nature wasn't known, and it was identified by the period of time between major attacks of fever. A quotidian fever struck every day, a tertian fever renewed its vigour on the third day, and a quartan fever on the fourth day. (This is now known to depend on the lifecycle of the *Plasmodium* species involved.)

Bloodletting aimed to draw off the fever and rebalance the humours, but it all came down to the patient hanging on in there and waiting for life or death to prevail.

Agostino Salumbrino (1561–1642), an Italian missionary equipped with the requisite zeal, travelled to Peru in 1605 to join the Jesuit community at San Pablo, Lima. The Jesuits had an infirmary there but it wasn't up to much and Salumbrino set to work establishing a pharmacy.

Peru already had a substantial materia medica – the Quechua people used a wide range of botanic substances including coca, from which cocaine would later be isolated. Historically, malaria had not been a problem for the Peruvian population, but Spain's colonisation of the region after its defeat of the Inca Empire in 1572 brought this Old World disease to new bloodstreams.

It's not clear whether the Quechua people used their existing pharmacopoeia to combat this threat, but somehow Salumbrino got the idea that a tree bark used to stop people shivering could also work for malarial chills. He sent some back to Rome in 1631. There, physicians found it remarkably effective, and from then on, whenever representatives returned to Rome from San Pablo, they carried as much 'Peruvian Bark' as they could squeeze into their luggage. Confusion arose about the name of the tree and the term 'quinquina' came into use, even though that was a different plant.

In 1742, the taxonomist Carl Linnaeus named the tree genus *Cinchona*, after the Countess of Chinchón (who had supposedly obtained a miraculous cure of her malaria and taken the bark back to Spain in the 1630s). Why Linnaeus left out the first 'h' is a mystery – maybe he'd had a long day – but as the Countess legend wasn't true anyway, it didn't matter.

Quinine – an active ingredient isolated from cinchona bark in 1820 – is no longer the primary treatment for malaria; it was replaced in the twentieth century by more effective medicines with fewer side effects. It remains, however, an important backup treatment. With malaria killing a child every minute in sub-Saharan Africa, and with *Plasmodium* starting to resist the first-line treatments, this 400-year-old medicine is in no danger of becoming obsolete.

48. The Iconic Plague Doctor Costume Protected Those Dealing with Pestilence

When the mysterious figure of the Medico della Peste turns its soulless round eyes and sinister curved beak towards you, you could be forgiven for fearing an immediate and agonising death from bubonic plague. The plague doctor, his identity concealed under a bird-like mask and long, dark coat, has become a cultural trope infecting diverse forms of entertainment from the Venetian *carnevale* to comic books.

There is no evidence that such a costume was prevalent during the fourteenth-century Black Death, but it did emerge in the seventeenth century. When plague rode in on its swirling miasma of doom, the outfit gave a sense of protection to those few doctors courageous enough to remain in town.

Its invention is usually credited to the French doctor Charles De Lorme (1584–1678), whose involvement with plague did not stop him living to the age of ninety-four and amassing fame and fortune as a promoter of spa towns, physician to the French monarchy, and provider of 'antimonyall cupps'. These cups, lined with antimony, were supposed to imbue wine with health-giving properties.

De Lorme did not leave any account of the plague doctor gear in his own words; it is linked to him by the theologian Michel de Saint-Martin, who published an account of De Lorme's career four years after the doctor's death. In *Moyens faciles et eprouves dont M. de l'Orme premier Medicin et ordinaire de trois de nos Rois,* Michel described the long morocco leather coat and the mask to which De Lorme attached 'a nose half a foot long to divert the malignant air'.

Such malignant air was the mainstay of miasma theory, which held that plague arose from poisonous vapours, affecting many individuals within the same locality at one time. Later accounts of the beak mask describe it as filled with perfumes and anointed inside with balsamic preparations.

Swiss physician Jean-Jacques Manget (1652–1742) included an illustration of the costume in his *Traité de la peste recueilli des meilleurs auteurs anciens et modernes,* written in 1721 after the plague of Marseilles. While he did not credit it to De Lorme, he stressed that it had been in use for a great many years and that the Italians employed similar designs.

Manget described the two holes in the beak, which would enable the wearer to breathe and also to take in the impression of the drugs carried within it. Under a long goatskin coat, the practitioner wore a leather shirt tucked into breeches, which in turn were tucked into boots. His hat and gloves were of the same leather. Contemporary representations also show the plague doctor carrying a stick with which to lift the patients' clothes and examine them from a distance.

The plague doctor might appear a frightening figure, bringing Death in his wake, but he also deserves credit for staying to help people in a situation where the easiest thing would be to flee.

49. THE CHAMBERLEN FAMILY WAS GOOD AT KEEPING SECRETS

Naming both your sons Peter saves time when calling them for dinner; beyond that, it just adds to the general confusion. This, however, was what Guillaume and Genevieve Chamberlen did in the late seventeenth century. As Huguenots – members of the French Protestant Church – they were in danger of slaughter during the Wars of Religion, so they fled to Southampton in 1569. Their sons, known as Peter the Elder (1560–1631) and Peter the Younger (1572–1626), grew up to become the guardians of a secret system of midwifery that they and their descendants concealed for more than a hundred years.

Both sons became barber-surgeons and 'accoucheurs' (man-midwives) and, towards the end of the sixteenth century, one of them (it's usually thought to be the older one) developed a design of obstetric forceps.

Most sixteenth-century births were uneventfully attended by female midwives, but when complications occurred, they were expected to send for a male surgeon – and such desperate circumstances called for desperate measures. Accoucheurs might have to use hooks to pull the baby out, or even remove it bit by bit in order to save the mother. The presence of a bloke in the birthing chamber therefore became associated with tragedy.

The new forceps were intended to increase the chances of both mother and baby surviving. They comprised two smoothly curved, fenestrated blades that could be positioned one at a time around the child's head and then joined together with a rivet or cord to operate with a scissor-like movement.

The Chamberlens did not, however, send their invention out into the world as a saviour of infants. For a century, only they and their descendants knew what it was, and as they successfully delivered countless royal and aristocratic babies, their prestige and fortune grew.

One of Peter the Younger's sons was called – wait for it – Peter. He achieved a medical degree in 1619 and is usually referred to as 'Dr Peter' to distinguish him from the previous generation. His father and uncle had unsuccessfully advocated for improvements to midwifery training, and Dr Peter (1601–83) attempted something similar, but neither the College of Physicians nor the midwives themselves were impressed with his plans to take charge of it. The latter accused Peter of lacking practical experience and gaining all his knowledge from books – for them, attending lots of deliveries and learning from other midwives was more effective than formal education.

The secret kept two further generations of Chamberlens in business, but by the time of the death of Dr Peter's grandson Hugh in 1728, it had begun to spread. The man-midwife was no longer a harbinger of death but a standard presence in the delivery room, further reducing the status of female midwifery. The Chamberlens' relationship to midwifery was ambiguous; supportive of attempts to improve the quality of training and form guilds, they ultimately undermined female midwives and instigated the medicalisation of childbirth. Another contradiction emerges from their close guarding of the invention – designed to save lives, the forceps were nevertheless kept secret for financial gain.

50. Midwives Protested Against Male Usurpers

The trend towards greater involvement of men in the birthing room threatened the traditional female midwife, who increasingly found herself marginalised in favour of surgeons. In 1671, Jane Sharp wrote a book that sought to defend her occupation from its takeover by men, to educate her sister midwives in anatomy, and to inform expectant mothers about pregnancy and childbirth. Midwifery manuals existed, but they were written by men. Sharp's *The Midwives Book* treated these precursors irreverently, never challenging them by name but casting sly references that would be picked up by those familiar with the other texts.

The Midwives Book covered the reproductive anatomy of both sexes and the mode of conception (subjects within the remit of the midwife's advice) in a candid, often witty tone. Sharp relied on the works of Nicholas Culpeper and Helkiah Crooke for her medical and anatomical information, but her own forthright and colloquial voice brought a lively humour to her subject. Writing of pregnancy cravings, she made fun of a gruesome current tale that a pregnant woman had eaten her spouse: 'She hath a preternatural desire to something not fit to eat nor drink, as some women with child have longed to bite off a piece of their Husbands Buttocks.' Advice on childbirth was reassuringly down to earth – once the waters had broken, she wrote, 'the Infant can no longer stay there than a naked man in a heap of snow.'

As the Chamberlens had discovered when they suggested improvements in training, midwives set great store by long years of practical experience rather than academic study. Sharp left no biographical detail other than to say she had been a midwife for thirty years at the time *The Midwives Book* came out. Later advertisements for the work upped this to forty years, from which one might speculate that she was still alive and practising in the early 1680s. She had probably learnt her craft by observing older practitioners; she believed midwifery was naturally the province of women, 'and though nature be not alone sufficient to the perfection of it, yet farther knowledge may be gain'd by a long and diligent practice, and be communicated to others of our own sex'.

In spite of the importance of experience, Sharp also knew that women's lack of formal educational opportunities was putting them at a disadvantage against surgeons who had access to anatomical texts. She was well aware that not all midwives were paragons of wisdom and experience – the unskilled among them would endanger women and fuel the stereotype of the ignorant midwife who had to call in a man when the going got tough. *The Midwives Book* aimed to supply the text-based knowledge her fellow midwives needed, and raise the skills level for the sake of both patients and female practitioners.

During the seventeenth and eighteenth centuries, British midwives did continue to lose their status to the new breed of 'man-midwife', but in *The Midwives Book* we see an educated, experienced midwife attempting to do something about it.

51. THE MICROSCOPE REVEALED A WHOLE NEW WORLD OF MINUSCULE LIFE

In Delft in the Netherlands in the 1670s, there arose a significant development for the history of medicine but, at the time, it had nothing to do with medicine. Antonie van Leeuwenhoek (1632–1723) observed creatures so tiny that millions of them danced in a single drop of water.

Van Leeuwenhoek was a textile merchant whose interest in the magnifying lenses used for inspecting cloth developed into a fascination for microscopes. He created hundreds of his own devices – tiny globes of glass, held firm between brass plates, with specimens mounted on a point that could be moved closer or further away by screws.

He corresponded with the Royal Society, London, whose secretary Henry Oldenburg (1619–77) encouraged the exchange of ideas with continental Europe. In 1674, one of his letters described a strange phenomenon. In a sample of lake water, he had seen 'very many little animalcules' of different colours and shapes, darting about in a manner 'wonderful to see'. These were protozoa; a longer letter in 1676 detailed observations of rain water, sea water and pepper-water, in which he saw creatures so 'incredibly small' that a hundred would not stretch to the width of a grain of sand. These were almost certainly bacteria.

The idea of millions of minuscule animals disporting themselves in every puddle was bizarre. It's now reminiscent of a Swiftian satire or the 1830s hoax about a civilisation on the moon. The Royal Society met Van Leeuwenhoek's discoveries with scepticism.

When looking back on the history of science and medicine, it's customary for some folks to revel in instances of villainous establishment figures scorning new developments. The Royal Society's caution, however, was warranted. You can't go around believing every wacky idea anyone throws at you. If, however, those wacky results can be replicated enough times to generate a consensus that they are accurate, everyone is happy.

The Royal Society did science. Oldenburg asked Van Leeuwenhoek to describe his method of viewing the animalcules, so others could repeat the experiments. Van Leeuwenhoek was cagey, going into detail about his preparation of the specimens but not about the construction of his microscopes, which he kept to himself for the rest of his life.

The Society commissioned the botanist and microscopist Nehemiah Grew (1641–1712) to look for the animalcules; he did not observe any. Robert Hooke (1635–1703), however, did manage to spot the creatures and on 15 November 1677, he successfully demonstrated them to the Royal Society's satisfaction.

Van Leeuwenhoek continued to fit scientific investigation around his business commitments, taking every opportunity for further discovery. When suffering from the trots in the summer of 1681, he even put his excrement under the microscope and saw flagellate protozoa that his biographer Christopher Dobell has identified as *Giardia intestinalis*, a cause of giardiasis, plus other microorganisms. This was the first indication that the human digestive system hosted millions of microscopic passengers. Van Leeuwenhoek did not link them to health and disease, but their importance to medicine would later become apparent.

52. THE FIRST PATENT MEDICINES INTRODUCED A NEW TREATMENT OPTION

In the early seventeenth century, a new phenomenon appeared in Europe – the newspaper. Published at regular intervals and collecting diverse news items in one convenient format, they took off rapidly and, as circulation grew, they became the perfect medium for advertising.

If someone invented a new medicine, newspapers were the place to tell everyone about it. In Britain, Anderson's Scots Pills (a mild laxative) and Daffy's Elixir (a 'health-bringing drink') were among the earliest medicines promoted in this way. Competition was rife, and the proprietors of successful remedies had to be on their guard against counterfeiters. Some (including Anthony Daffy, successor to the Elixir's inventor) printed vitriolic name-and-shame attacks against their imitators, but to little effect.

Others, like Southwark apothecary Richard Stoughton, sought a more official means of protecting their right as sole manufacturer. After about twenty years selling Stoughton's Elixir for all indispositions of the stomach, he received the third English medicinal patent in 1712 (the first two were for products still instantly recognisable – Epsom Salts in 1698 and Sal Volatile in 1711).

As well as protecting the medicines' formulae, royal patents became another marketing tool. Advertisements headed 'By Authority of the King's Royal Patent' had an impressive ring to them and while they did not explicitly claim that the King himself used the medicine, it was all well and good if people happened to believe that. The term 'patent medicine' soon came to mean any advertised remedy, even though the vast majority were never patented.

During the eighteenth century, British emigrants to America took commercial medicines with them and, although the British brands predominated at first, American entrepreneurs soon took advantage of the market. Patent medicines became big business on both sides of the pond and their exaggerated claims and secret ingredients made them synonymous with quackery.

By keeping the formulae secret, vendors could claim that they contained something new, for example herbs from a distant land that would supersede the limited pharmacopoeia of the humdrum doctor. This was a good reason not to patent the remedy, which would require an open specification of how to make it. In practice, the formulae tended to be unremarkable, and differed little from the prescriptions of qualified physicians.

Patent medicines were cheap – or at least cheaper than consulting a doctor, and in isolated areas there might not even be a doctor to consult. They were easily available from the local newspaper office, grocery shop or by post from the cities. They were discreet; an embarrassing ailment need not be disclosed in person. Advertisements promised a swift and painless effect compared with the harsh remedies associated with regular physicians. Although the industry acquired a dubious reputation and became home to fraudsters just looking for a quick buck, there were many reasons for patients to see advertised medicines as an attractive option.

53. Smallpox Inoculation Reached England via Constantinople

In 1722, an excoriating essay appeared in the British newspaper *The Flying Post*. 'A Plain Account of the Inoculating of the Smallpox by a Turkey Merchant' castigated physicians for incorrectly adopting the Turkish practice of smallpox inoculation. By their overzealous adaptations to traditional methods, they were endangering people's lives.

The author was later identified as Lady Mary Wortley Montagu (1689–1762), whose determination to make inoculation popular in England began when she encountered the practice in Constantinople. Smallpox inoculation, already widespread in China, the Middle East and Africa, conferred immunity from a disease that was at best disfiguring and at worst deadly. It would, however, prove controversial, and the 'Plain Account' was part of a heated exchange of views between supporters and opponents.

In a letter to Sarah Chiswell in 1717, Lady Mary described the procedure: '… the old woman comes with a nutshell full of the best sort of small-pox and asks what veins you please to have opened. She immediately rips open that you offer her with a large needle (which gives you no more pain than a common scratch) and puts into the vein as much venom as can lye upon the head of her needle …' The patient would suffer a mild case of smallpox but, once recovered, would have immunity for life.

When Lady Mary returned to England in 1718, having had her son inoculated in Turkey, the practice was not entirely unknown to the medical profession. The *Philosophical Transactions of the Royal Society* had published two communications about it within the past few years. These accounts, however, did not make any difference to the general population, who continued to suffer the disease. Lady Mary might have used the language of frivolity when she signified her intent to 'bring this useful invention into fashion', but high-profile examples were exactly what was needed to raise awareness of the procedure. When a smallpox epidemic gripped Britain in 1721, Lady Mary's three-year-old daughter became the first person inoculated by a member of the medical profession in England. Word began to spread, and other members of high society followed the example.

The practice also met with opposition – not least because smallpox could be fatal and it seemed counterintuitive to infect one's loved ones. Then there was the argument that only God had authority to inflict disease; the fact that inoculation was foreign and therefore probably a bit suspect; and, in the words of William Wagstaffe, physician to Barts Hospital, that it was '... an experiment practised only by a few *Ignorant Women*, amongst an illiterate and unthinking people ...'

Fortunately, one of those Ignorant Women happened to be the Princess of Wales, and she had the influential royal physician, Sir Hans Sloane, on her side. In August 1721, Sloane supervised one of the earliest known clinical trials, an experiment at Newgate Gaol, where six prisoners had agreed to undergo inoculation in return for a pardon. After further tests on parish orphans, Princess Caroline was convinced of the procedure's safety and had her daughters inoculated on 18 April 1722. Such a celebrity endorsement helped bring inoculation into fashion.

54. ... And Arrived in America from Africa ...

Smallpox inoculation began in America at about the same time as it reached England. The practice, however, arrived via a different route that suggests a long history of inoculation in African medicine.

An enslaved man, given the name Onesimus by the Reverend Cotton Mather of Boston, described having been inoculated against smallpox. He answered 'Yes and no' to the question of whether he had ever been infected, and went on to describe the procedure and the principles behind it.

Onesimus' exact country of origin is unknown, but other Africans in Boston were familiar with the practice too, implying that it was not confined to a single community. One man interviewed by pro-inoculation campaigner Benjamin Colman explained that in his home country, inoculation was useful for merchants – it enabled them to travel hundreds of miles on business without fear of contracting smallpox along the way. Inoculation had been around so long that he didn't know how it originated.

Opposition to inoculation in colonial Boston was even greater than that in England, and the newspapers were bombarded with angry letters accusing supporters of being 'infatuated' with the idea of infecting healthy people. Underlying the criticism was a difficulty with accepting that African medical knowledge could introduce such an important means of tackling a deadly disease – the whole concept undermined the justifications for enslaving a supposedly inferior race. Only about six hundred people were inoculated during the 1721 epidemic, but when the death rate in that group was just 2 per cent, compared with 14 per cent among those infected naturally, public opinion began to change.

55. ... AND THEN VACCINATION BECAME POSSIBLE

Inoculation became widespread in Britain, especially after the 1760s when safer methods were introduced. The practice revealed an interesting phenomenon – a lot of people in farming communities did not come down with the expected mild case of smallpox. A vague idea took shape that this applied to those who'd had cowpox in the past, and at the end of the eighteenth century, Edward Jenner's scientific approach to this knowledge led to the development of vaccination.

In 1838, Jenner's biographer, James Baron, related the story of a young countrywoman who said of smallpox: 'I cannot take that disease, for I have had cowpox.' This was supposed to have inspired Jenner on a heroic quest. Jenner himself, however, never mentioned such an incident and it is likely that Baron embellished the reality. Later writers turned the woman into a milkmaid and added the fairytale-like detail that cowpox had saved her from having an ugly pockmarked face. Such 'Eureka moments' are compelling, but it's probably just a story.

Jenner (1749–1823) did not claim to have discovered the cowpox–smallpox correlation – he might have heard about it from Gloucester surgeon John Fewster, who in turn learnt it from farmers and reported it to a local medical society in 1768. What Jenner did do, however, was scientifically test the validity of these ideas and develop a person-to-person procedure that did away with the dangers of inoculation.

Looking back from 1801, Jenner remembered: 'I was struck with the idea that it might be practicable to propagate the disease by inoculation, after the manner of the Small Pox, first from the Cow, and finally from one human being to another.'

Obstacles beset him – some people who said they'd had cowpox turned out to be susceptible to smallpox after all. Jenner realised this was because the term 'cowpox' could apply to all manner of random bovine pustules. Even the genuine cowpox could fail to make people smallpox-immune if they caught it during its later stages. He spent decades learning about the disease and the point at which infection would most reliably confer immunity. In the meantime, someone did try using cowpox (direct from the cow) for inoculation. In 1774, Gloucestershire farmer Benjamin Jesty deliberately infected members of his family, with the result that they stayed healthy through later smallpox epidemics. In the face of local hostility, however, Jesty did nothing to disseminate the procedure, waiting until Jenner became famous before he popped up with a priority claim.

Jenner, however, put his hypothesis to the test by conducting an experiment. In May 1796 he vaccinated a boy called James Phipps with matter from a cowpox pustule on the hand of a milkmaid, Sarah Nelmes. Seven weeks later, and again after several months, he inoculated Phipps with proper smallpox – no disease followed.

Jenner published his results in 1798, calling his procedure 'vaccination' (from *vacca*, the Latin word for cow). Although he encountered initial opposition, vaccination soon replaced inoculation as the standard means of smallpox prevention, and later gave its name to vaccines protecting against many other diseases.

56. Germany's First Female MD Championed Women's Education

More than four hundred years after Jacoba Felicie's conviction (see Fact 31), universities remained closed to women, apart from in very rare cases. In 1754, Dorothea Erxleben was the first woman in Germany to gain a medical degree, but even her success did not set a precedent for women's entry into the profession. Her experience shows how it was necessary for circumstances to align in order for one individual to access the opportunities denied to her gender as a whole.

Erxleben (1715–62) was born Dorothea Christiane Leporin in Quedlinburg. In an autobiographical note appended to her dissertation, she described how childhood illness proved to be positive for her – her father, a doctor, allowed her to study alongside her brother in order to take her mind off her troubles. Education turned out to be a treatment for her illness, just as she would come to see it as a remedy for women's situation in society.

Her health improving as she grew up, Erxleben acquired her medical knowledge via an informal apprenticeship to her father. She used his difficult cases as examples for working out treatment regimes, and sometimes attended patients on his behalf. In 1740, she petitioned Frederick II of Prussia to allow her admittance to the university of Halle, where her brother intended to go. The king granted her request and Erxleben began her studies in 1742. They were cut short, however, when her brother was called up to the army and she felt it inappropriate to remain at Halle alone.

Back in Quedlinburg, she married pastor Johann Erxleben, becoming stepmother to his five children. Like her father, he was an advocate for the Enlightenment value of equality and supported her as she built up a medical practice. She was writing too – her *Thorough Investigation into the Causes that Prevent Women from Studying* appeared in 1742, encouraging women to take responsibility for their own education, and not to fall into the stereotype of being too emotional to use their innate reason. Any lack of control over the emotions, she argued, was the consequence of exclusion from education, not a reason to perpetuate that exclusion.

As an unqualified practitioner, and a female one at that, she was subjected to a negative campaign by three local physicians, who complained that 'quacks' like her were making it impossible for licensed doctors to make a living. In 1753, after the death of a patient, they accused her of malpractice. As Erxleben argued, 'let the doctor who has never had a patient die cast the first stone', but this rebuttal of gendered double standards made little impression on her opponents. Public officials ordered her to take a university exam in order to continue practising. She was, however, about to give birth, so she had the baby first and did the exam the following year, passing and receiving her medical degree. She practised as a doctor in Quedlinburg until her death eight years later.

Despite this, Erxleben's experience did not lead to an influx of women into the medical profession. It was 1908 before Prussian universities officially granted them entry.

57. A Self-Help Manual Taught That Cleanliness Was Key

To whom do you turn in the middle of the night when a child is feverish, darkness magnifies fears, the nearest doctor is miles away and, anyway, there's no money for his fee? In the late eighteenth and early nineteenth centuries, whether you were in Scotland or Russia, Germany or America, in a city tenement or a remote farm, you always had Dr William Buchan by your side.

Buchan (1729–1805), a Scottish physician, published *Domestic Medicine* in 1769. Medical handbooks aimed at ordinary people were not new, but Buchan's was to become a household name in Europe and America, running to more than twenty editions and numerous translations. In an engaging style, he set out to empower people with knowledge of health and disease.

Domestic Medicine contained formulae for ointments, plasters and syrups, but it wasn't first and foremost a medical recipe book. Its advice focused on prevention of disease through lifestyle and hygiene, emphasising cleanliness of the body and the environment. A simple diet, outdoor exercise, frequent washing and clean clothes all contributed to health and, importantly, they were positive things individuals could do for themselves and their families.

Infection control was paramount, even though Buchan was not aware of the exact mode of disease transmission. In *Domestic Medicine*, the ideas of humours, miasma and contagion lived happily alongside one another. Diseases could come from the air, which picked up aspects of any decaying or filthy matter it touched. They could also pass from one person to another on clothing and possessions; it was dangerous to 'buy at random the clothes which have been worn by other people'. Buchan advised staying away from ill people apart from to give them the necessary care and comfort. Nosy neighbours crowding into the sick person's house would just make everything worse, disturbing the patient and taking disease away with them. He recommended that all who cared for the sick should change their clothes and wash their hands before coming into contact with anyone else.

As well as disease, Buchan dealt with the common experiences of life, from emotional difficulties to childbirth to hangovers. (Water and toast were best for the latter, but staying sober in the first place was preferable.) Buchan advocated wider public health measures too – he was a proponent of smallpox inoculation, hospital hygiene and wholesome water supplies, and suggested that, ideally, the streets of towns should be washed every day. He was aware that, although the individual could do a lot to improve their own situation, public leaders should be taking responsibility for improving sanitation.

Buchan has been described as 'ahead of his time' for his sensible advice on infection control, but he was an eighteenth-century doctor talking to eighteenth-century people in the eighteenth century; he cannot be of any time but his own. *Domestic Medicine*'s popularity makes it an important source of information on how families and communities approached the issues of health and disease.

58. Bloodletting Was a Perennial Favourite

The unhappy chap on the cover of this book is undergoing bloodletting, a procedure widespread across many cultures. He's from the first of a series of prints by British artist James Gillray, who satirised the bleedings, emetics and laxatives that constituted the medical treatment of his time. The character ends up 'Charming Well Again' despite all this intervention.

Gillray caricatured bloodletting in 1804, but by then the procedure had been around for thousands of years. The ancient Ayurvedic *Sushruta Samhita* went into detail about it. The Hippocratic writers acknowledged bloodletting but didn't go overboard, while Galen was more enthusiastic – his theory that blood travelled in one direction to the extremities provided a rationale for getting rid of an accumulation. Bloodletting remained popular (with patients as well as doctors) until the late Victorian era, when it receded from practise. It is now only used in a few specific cases, such as haemochromatosis, a genetic condition causing a build-up of iron in the blood.

The goal of bloodletting was to balance the four humours. As the most active humour, blood could become dominant, leaving the others struggling to assert themselves. Removing some blood took it back to its rightful quantity and promoted equilibrium. It therefore applied to all sorts of ailments.

In the mid-eighteenth century, a distinction still prevailed between physicians and surgeons. Although surgeons' status had improved, they remained the handymen of the medical world. The physician prescribed bloodletting; the surgeon carried it out. Although leeches were used for the most delicate patients, the most common method was venesection – cutting the vein with a sharp blade.

Blood could be let from a variety of locations including the temples, the veins under the tongue, and even the penis, but the standard place for venesection was the inside of the forearm, near the elbow joint. The surgeon wrapped a cloth ligature round the upper arm to slow the circulation and make the veins more visible. He could pick from the cephalic, basilic and median veins, depending on which looked the nicest. The surgeon pressed his thumb onto the vein to make it more prominent, then pushed a lancet forwards and upwards into the vein. The usual practice was to make an oblique cut, but it wasn't a disaster if you did a straight one. It was important neither to be too gung-ho nor too reticent about this. Slashing away willy-nilly was likely to damage the nerves or tendons (which you would know about when the patient leapt up and punched you in the face), but squeamishness and faffiness wouldn't get the job done, either.

After bloodletting, once the arm was cleaned up and bandaged, and the patient's strength revived with a glass of wine, came perhaps the most important part of the whole operation – a positive prognosis. German surgical authority Lorenz Heister emphasised the need to promote 'the good effects that follow, from cheering the patient's mind'. The eighteenth-century surgeon was well aware of how to exploit placebo responses even before the idea of the 'placebo' had fully taken shape.

59. Tractors Demonstrated the Placebo Effect

Eighteenth-century Bath was a magnet for people of fashion. Assemblies, coffee houses, theatre and dance; sulphuric health-giving waters and Pump Rooms gossip, it was the perfect hothouse for the latest fad. At the close of the century, an American invention called Perkins' Metallic Tractors became the talk of the town.

The Tractors originated with Connecticut physician Elisha Perkins (1741–99), who patented them in 1796. These tapered metal prongs drew on the ideas of the Italian physician Luigi Galvani, who postulated that the body contained a fluid analogous to electricity. Perkins believed this fluid could bunch up in the body, causing pain. Drawing the Tractors over the skin would smooth it out.

Benjamin Perkins, son of Elisha, took the Tractors to England in 1798. Promotional material recommended them for rheumatism, eye inflammation, boils, epilepsy and many other complaints. The Tractors became fashionable in Bath, home of John Haygarth (1740–1827), who had just retired there after a distinguished career as a physician in Chester.

Haygarth was sceptical about the Tractors but prepared to accept they might work. He wrote to William Falconer, physician at Bath Infirmary, proposing an impartial test. Haygarth and Falconer constructed wooden Tractors, painted to resemble the real thing. They then conducted a single-blind trial where the doctor performing the procedure knew the devices were counterfeit, but the patients didn't.

The experiments started on 7 January 1799. Five patients with chronic rheumatism underwent treatment with the fake Tractors. Three felt a significant improvement and one gained some relief. The fifth, whose condition was not painful to start with, reported no change. The following day, Haygarth and Falconer used real Tractors, and the patients had a similar response. Haygarth concluded that this showed 'what powerful Influence upon diseases is produced by mere imagination'.

The word 'placebo' (literally 'I shall please') had appeared in a medical context in recent decades. In 1772, William Cullen used it to describe a medicine given to encourage the patient when there was little hope of curative effects. Haygarth himself did not use the term, but his experiments did show what we would now recognise as placebo effects – i.e. those resulting from something other than a physiological response to the treatment.

'The placebo effect', however, was not (and still isn't), a single thing. Many factors can combine to change someone's perception of their pain. Belief in the treatment can cause the production of endorphins; then there's the patient's desire to get better, their wish to leave the hospital, their faith in the stories of wonderful cures, and so on. As a single-blind trial, Haygarth's experiments probably included some reporting bias on the part of the experimenters, too.

Haygarth published his results in 1800 in *Of the imagination, as a cause and as a cure of disorders of the body*. He concluded that the Metallic Tractors could not be operating on the principle of Galvanic electricity. More importantly, he pointed out that if the trials hadn't included the pretend Tractors, the real ones would have appeared impressive – he was illustrating the importance of comparing new treatments against a control.

60. GENERAL ANAESTHESIA ALLAYED THE PAIN OF CANCER SURGERY

Kan Aiya, a sixty-year-old woman, had lost her sisters to breast cancer, so when she found a lump, she was well aware of the likely outcome. For her, however, there was a chance of survival – an operation. It was 1804 and she was in the best possible place for surgery – feudal Japan.

Seishu Hanaoka (1760–1835) had studied Chinese medicine in Kyoto and set up a practice in his hometown of Hirayama. The Tokugama Shogunate had expelled all foreign traders from Japan in 1639, with the exception of the Dutch, who were permitted to trade in Nagasaki. Through this conduit, bits and pieces of outside influence, including medical information, reached interested parties like Hanaoka. His surgical practice combined Chinese and Dutch methods.

Hanaoka became interested in anaesthesia owing to stories that a third-century Chinese surgeon, Houa T'o, had developed a drug enabling patients to sleep through pain. Hanaoka experimented with similar formulae and produced *tsusentan,* a potent hot drink. It contained *Datura metel*, a source of scopolamine, atropine and hyoscamine – plus five other botanical ingredients. Tsusentan had quite a kick and if you glugged it down haphazardly you would probably die, but in the correct dosage it rendered patients unconscious for between six and twenty-four hours, allowing ample time for surgery.

On 13 October 1804, Hanaoka excised Kan Aiya's tumour while she was under general anaesthesia, going on to operate on at least 150 more breast cancer patients. Kan Aiya sadly died of her disease the following year, but had been spared the agony that still characterised surgery outside Japan.

61. Smoking Was Good for You

The words 'cigarettes' and 'health' are now unlikely bedfellows. Nineteenth-century medical cigarettes for asthma, however, were part of a long history of inhalation therapy that evolved over centuries and continues its legacy today.

Ancient systems of medicine interpreted asthma within the context of the four humours. The condition was thought to result from a build up of phlegm in the lungs; it made sense to send treatment directly to the site of the problem. Inhalation of the smoke of burning herbs would enable the phlegm to dissipate. After the medieval period, ideas about asthma began to change, putting more emphasis on it as a whole-body disease involving the stomach and other organs; under this interpretation, inhalation fell out of favour. During the eighteenth century, however, inhalation came back as an efficient way of getting medicines into the respiratory system, and new inhaler designs made administering treatment easier. Ideas about asthma changed again and by the end of the century it was becoming known as a 'nervous' disease caused by spasms of the bronchi.

Into this receptive medical environment came the plant *Datura stramonium*, or thorn-apple (a relative of Hanaoka's anaesthetic herb). Already known in the US, it appeared in Britain between 1802 and 1810, after a similar remedy, *Datura ferox*, was brought back by one of the East India Company's physicians. Joseph Toulmin, a surgeon from Hackney, substituted the more easily obtainable *D. stramonium*, gaining relief from his own asthma, and word quickly spread that there was a new remedy in town.

At first, stramonium was smoked in ordinary tobacco

pipes. It was possible to grow it oneself and prepare the roots and stalks (not the leaves, which have a dangerous narcotic effect) by drying them, brushing off the mould and chopping them into small pieces.

By the middle of the nineteenth century smoking was socially acceptable, manly, and ever easier with the introduction of cigars, then cigarettes (and matches, too). Henry Hyde Salter, a leading authority on asthma, advocated ordinary tobacco as a cure for asthma attacks. In his 1864 book, *On Asthma, Its Pathology and Treatment*, Salter discussed stramonium too, advising its regular use as a preventive. By this time, ready-prepared stramonium cigarettes were available over the counter and were recommended by doctors as a convenient way of inhaling the drug.

In the early twentieth century the spasmodic model of asthma gave way to the concept of allergic inflammation, and this made smoking seem less appropriate. At the same time, new drugs such as ephedrine were emerging, providing an alternative to the potentially hallucinogenic stramonium. As the dangers of tobacco smoking became more apparent, it became awkward for doctors to recommend medicated cigarettes. Changes in cultural attitudes to smoking, along with new drugs and inhalers (e.g. salbutamol in 1969), saw stramonium disappear from the arsenal against asthma – but it had played an important role in bringing relief to those struggling to breathe.

62. A MUTINEER LED IMPROVEMENTS IN CONVICT HEALTH

William Redfern (*c.* 1774–1833) didn't get very far in his career as a ship's surgeon. Newly qualified in 1797, he enlisted as surgeon's mate on the Royal Navy's HMS Standard. In May that year, however, the crew participated in the fleet-wide Nore Mutiny, taking over the ship in protest against pay arrears. Redfern, who allegedly encouraged the men to stay united, was considered a ringleader and sentenced to death. After a reprieve and four years in prison, he was transported to Sydney in December 1801.

From the early seventeenth century until 1776, Britain had been sending convicted felons to the American colonies. With America declaring independence, however, the government needed new territory on which to dump its undesirables. The penal colony of New South Wales, in what would soon become known as Australia, received its founding members in January 1788. Transportation remained a sentencing option until 1868, by which time more than 162,000 convicts had made the journey.

Redfern's inelegant exit from Britain did not detract from his talents as a surgeon. As well as treating fellow convicts on the voyage over, he was soon appointed assistant surgeon to Norfolk Island, and in 1803 received a free pardon, going on to run the Sydney Hospital for convicts and develop an extensive private practice.

Convict ships were crowded and insanitary. The government expected the odd death on the way but, in 1814, three catastrophic voyages stood out. The *General Hewitt* lost thirty-four of its 300 convicts; the *Three Bees* lost ten out of 220, and the *Surry* lost thirty-six out of 200, plus more deaths among the crew – including the ship's surgeon. Typhus and scurvy were the main culprits. The Governor of New South Wales, Major-General Lachlan Macquarie (1762–1824), commissioned Redfern to report on the causes of this loss of life and how to stop it happening again.

Redfern recommended that sanitation facilities be improved, warm clothes provided, convicts and their bedding allowed on deck for air, the ships to be fumigated with nitric acid and for everyone to get their full ration of food. His most significant recommendation was that each ship should have a principal medical officer authorised to enforce the sanitary rules. In his view, ships' surgeons were either lacking in experience or jaded old drunks with little authority to stand up to bullying captains.

As a result of Redfern's report, a new system of 'surgeon-superintendents' was introduced – experienced Royal Navy surgeons who held responsibility for the health of the convicts on board. They treated illness, but also preserved health by checking the quality of provisions, overseeing cleanliness and fumigations, ensuring the convicts were issued with warm clothes and that they took their rations of wine and lime juice against scurvy.

Mortality rates dropped and the journey to Australia was no longer something to be dreaded. The more conditions improved, the more people started travelling there willingly; transportation was no deterrent to crime and the thriving Australian settlements were increasingly resistant to having more criminals foisted on them. The last convict ship arrived in Fremantle, Western Australia, in January 1868.

63. A Paper Tube Became a Window to the Human Body

When a small child plays at being a doctor, it's perhaps fortunate that the dressing up kit does not contain a plastic urine bottle, ready to be waved under the dog in the hope of getting a sample. Although the urine bottle, or *matula*, was once symbolic of the medical profession, it has given way to another diagnostic tool – the stethoscope. The stethoscope was invented in 1816 by French physician René Théophile-Hyacinthe Laennec (1781–1826), who accompanied the device's development with an important treatise on the diseases of the lungs.

Prior to 1816, there were two useful but inadequate ways of working out what was going on inside a patient's chest. Percussion – tapping in different places and assessing the level of resonance – could reveal fluid in the lungs. Immediate auscultation – placing the ear directly against the chest – also gave away the telltale sounds of heart and lung conditions. It could, however, be awkward. With female patients, such intimacy was inappropriate, not to mention impractical for the larger bosomed. Some folk also had less-than-scrupulous attention to hygiene, which made the experience rather unpleasant for the more refined of physicians.

In late 1816, Laennec was consulted by a young woman with symptoms of heart disease. According to Laennec's own account, her 'great degree of fatness' made percussion useless, and immediate auscultation would have been indelicate. He remembered that if you put one ear to a wooden pole and scratch the other end with a pin, the sound is amplified. With this in mind, he rolled up a quire of paper and listened to the patient's chest through that, finding the heartbeat much more distinct.

He realised this could be a way of identifying other diseases too.

Laennec worked at the Hôpital Necker in Paris, and there he began testing different materials for the new instrument. He found that a foot-long wooden cylinder, with a funnel-shaped aperture down its length, worked best. His design divided in two for portability, and was furnished with a plug to close the aperture in cases where a solid cylinder was required. Laennec coined the term 'stethoscope' from the Greek words *stethos* (chest) and *skopein* (look at).

The stethoscope itself, however, could not tell the doctor what was wrong – it was necessary to develop the skill to recognise the sounds characterising each disease. The hospital environment was ideal for this; when patients died, autopsy could confirm the diagnosis. Laennec established the art of stethoscopy and presented his findings in *De l'Auscultation Médiate* (*On Mediate Auscultation*) in 1819. (Writing the book nearly killed him. Tell me about it, René.) Although a few critics made fun of the stethoscope, calling it 'Laennec's trumpetter', most of the medical profession immediately recognised its importance.

A revised second edition of *De l'Auscultation Médiate* appeared in 1826 and, again, the work took its toll on the author's health. Laennec's nephew, also a doctor, listened to his chest through the stethoscope and diagnosed pulmonary tuberculosis – one of the diseases that he had done so much to elucidate. He died in August 1826 at the age of forty-five.

64. BODYSNATCHERS HELPED STUDENTS LEARN ANATOMY

Two nights after Christmas 1796, a Hackney coachman snored in a cell at the New Prison, Clerkenwell, as he waited to go before the magistrate. Sharing his temporary accommodation were two men and three children. Their presence, however, did not disturb him, for they too slept the sleep of the dead ... literally.

The coachman had been caught dead-handed when his bodysnatcher employers scarpered from the Pesthouse burial ground in Old Street, leaving him with a coach full of cadavers. He was part of a growing trade in corpses, supplying London's anatomy schools with subjects for students to dissect.

Since 1752, anatomists had been allowed to dissect executed felons, but there weren't enough to go round. Bodysnatchers – called resurrection-men – supplied this deficit by exhuming the just-buried and selling them to the anatomy schools.

To steal a body, it wasn't worth digging up the whole grave; a small area at the head end sufficed. The resurrection-men levered up a portion of the coffin lid, snapping it back against the heavy soil, and dragged the corpse out by the head in a macabre parody of birth. As demand for corpses rose in the early nineteenth century, resurrection-men could charge whatever they liked; in 1828, when the government appointed a Select Committee to investigate the problems of cadaver supply, the going rate was eight to ten guineas per body.

The general public was outraged by bodysnatching and its gruesome bedfellow, dissection. Some had religious concerns about not being intact on Judgement Day, but the more immediate issue was the indignity of being cut up in a lecture theatre or joked over by irreverent students.

Surgeons were under no illusion that the resurrectionists had any scruples whatsoever. They were an essential evil. Sir Astley Cooper (1768–1841), president of the Royal College of Surgeons in London and keen purchaser of corpses, described them as 'the lowest dregs of degradation', but without them surgeons couldn't learn their job; patients would suffer.

By 1828, the legal situation had become confusing. The RCS would not licence a surgeon unless he had certificates of attendance at anatomy classes. An alternative path to qualification, the exams of Apothecaries' Hall, also required a thorough knowledge of anatomy. Yet having a cadaver in your possession put you on sketchy ground with the law. Something needed to be done, and the Select Committee considered allowing the dissection of unclaimed bodies from hospitals and workhouses. This could not be to anyone's detriment because the deceased had no relatives (or none who cared) and, in the words of Benjamin Brodie (1783–1862) of St George's Hospital, dissection 'cannot matter to the poor dead carcase.'

The Bill resulting from the 1828 Select Committee was withdrawn but, partly in response to the case of Burke and Hare, who murdered people to sell, the Anatomy Act was passed in 1832. It provided for the donation of cadavers in exchange for burial costs, and gave anatomists access to unclaimed bodies from institutions. The resurrection-men could no longer command their extortionate fees and moved on to other unsavoury schemes.

65. LEECHES WERE ALL THE RAGE

The medicinal leech has accompanied humankind through its travails for thousands of years. Always there to lend a healing hand, it nevertheless did not hit the big time until the early nineteenth century, when it became the worm of the moment – first in France and then in the rest of western Europe and America.

Led by François-Joseph-Victor Broussais (1772–1838), who postulated that all disease stemmed from local inflammation treatable by leeches, the 'leech craze' saw barrels of the creatures shipped across the world, and wild leech populations decimated almost to extinction.

The leech had advantages over the lancet. It took its time, gently drawing out blood without any heroics or mess. People considered too delicate to withstand venesection could benefit from the leech's careful suction. Leeches also made it possible to do targeted bloodletting in hard-to-reach places, including the anus and vagina (the surgeon had to put the leech on a little thread leash to stop it going on too much of an adventure). As a home remedy, leeches were unlikely to kill you, whereas an amateur attempt at bleeding someone with a knife could go disastrously wrong.

Traditionally, leech-collectors harvested the animals from ponds by wading in and waiting for them to attack, but as demand grew an international trade sprang up. German and Hungarian leeches found themselves aboard ship, going as far afield as the US, where the native leech species were less bitey. Doctors (or anyone, for that matter) could buy leeches from their local pharmacist, or direct from an importer such as Surgeon Daly in 1850s Belfast. Like many wholesalers and retailers, he advertised them with the catchy strapline 'LEECHES! LEECHES!! LEECHES!!!'

Brits were somewhat suspicious of French things, but the benefits of leech bleeding overcame objections. In 1822, a doctor called Rees Price published a treatise explaining how and when to use leeches. He called the therapy *sangui-suction*, a name that did not catch on at the time but could be the perfect new health fad should you feel like buying a PhD and setting up a fancy website. He detailed over ninety conditions in which leeches were of use, including typhus, gonorrhoea and scrofula.

Employing a leech wasn't just a case of plonking it on the patient and hoping for the best; the leeches didn't always have a strong work ethic and might require some persuasion to bite. Price recommended that the area of skin was cleared of hair and washed with soap and water. It could be moistened with milk, but he found porter the best thing for encouraging reluctant leeches. He applied them in an upturned wineglass; it was also possible to buy specialised glass tubes to direct the animal to the right place.

Leeching declined after the middle of the nineteenth century, but our little aquatic buddies didn't abandon us forever. Now produced on high-tech farms, they have an important role in overcoming venous congestion in graft tissue, and remain the doctor's colleagues in the pursuit of healing.

66. Elizabeth Fry Laid the Foundations for Nursing Reform

The Quaker philanthropist Elizabeth Fry (1780–1845), who appeared on the Bank of England's five pound note from 2002 to 2016, is remembered as an activist for prison reform. She campaigned to improve the appalling conditions facing women in prison – first at London's Newgate and later across Britain and Europe.

Among Fry's other achievements, however, were the first steps towards organising nursing as a profession. Early nineteenth-century nursing had a terrible reputation and was not something that anyone with other options would want to do. While many hospital nurses did work harder and pick up more clinical knowledge than they were given credit for, they had no formalised training, experienced poor working and living conditions, and were vulnerable to sexual harassment from patients and male hospital staff. Nursing was not, therefore, considered 'respectable'.

In 1840, when she was sixty years old and already becoming infirm, Fry set out to change this.

She was inspired by her friend Theodor Fliedner (1800–64), whose Kaiserswerth Diakonie in Düsseldorf trained young women as deaconesses to care for the sick in their community. (It was at Kaiserswerth that Florence Nightingale would later train.) After visiting Fliedner in May 1840, Fry set up an organisation called the Protestant Sisters of Charity, which aimed to provide competent and respectable uniformed nurses to care for patients in their own homes. In spite of the word 'Protestant', the name proved too reminiscent of Catholic religious orders and was changed in 1842 to the Institution of Nursing Sisters.

The women had up to three months of informal training

in one of the London teaching hospitals, shadowing the nurses and gaining practical experience. They were then employed to look after patients privately – those who could afford to pay did so, while the poor received care free of charge. Crucially, the 'Fry sisters' had a safe and comfortable environment in which to live, a nurses' home where they received full board and did not suffer the unwanted attentions of the various unsavouries who wandered about in hospitals.

Fry's personal attitude to nursing reflected the inner struggles she experienced throughout her life. When called upon to care for sick relatives, Fry was efficient and caring, but admitted in her diary that nursing was not her vocation. She found it painful to see people suffering, and her 'cheerful countenance' hid feelings of unworthiness and self-doubt. Similar anxieties underscored all her philanthropy; she relied on opium and port wine to assuage them, battling conflicts within herself while taking on society.

Her institution remained small and did not have the capacity to overhaul hospital nursing, but it began to change attitudes towards nurses and show the importance of clinical knowledge, good working conditions and the expectation of mutual respect between nurses, patients and doctors.

67. The Early Days of Inhalational Anaesthesia Were Hilarious ... and Tragic

'As nitrous oxide', wrote Humphry Davy in 1800, 'in its extensive operation appears capable of destroying physical pain, it may probably be used with advantage during surgical operations in which no great effusion of blood takes place.'

It was a profound observation, but neither Davy (later of mining lamp fame) nor anyone else developed the idea. They had more pressing concerns – namely, getting high. Davy (1778–1829) had been investigating nitrous oxide (laughing gas) in chemical and recreational detail, collecting his friends' accounts of their experiences under its influence. Samuel Taylor Coleridge (of Kubla Khan fame) felt a sensation like that 'after returning from a walk in the snow into a warm room'; Thomas Wedgwood (son of Josiah, of plate fame), felt 'a very strong inclination to make odd antic motions'. Peter Roget (of thesaurus fame), was less moved, stating 'I cannot remember that I experienced the least pleasure from any of these sensations.'

For more than forty years, nitrous oxide became a party drug, administered at private gatherings and public entertainments, where audiences delighted in the capers of the volunteers on stage.

Attending a demonstration by showman Gardner Quincey Colton in December 1844, Horace Wells (1815–48) observed that one participant injured himself without noticing. Wells was a dentist, concerned about his patients' pain, and he saw the gas's potential to assuage it. He tested it by having one of his own teeth extracted, and started employing the gas with excellent results in his practice in Hartford, Connecticut. In January 1845, he travelled to Boston, where he discussed the matter with his former business associate, William G. Morton (1819–68). While there, he arranged a public demonstration of his discovery – he would pull out a tooth and the patient wouldn't feel a thing.

The demonstration went pear-shaped. The patient didn't receive enough gas and experienced pain. To the audience, it was a ridiculous anti-climax; Wells looked a right idiot.

He was so mortified that he never really recovered. He became ill and unable to continue his dental practice. Things got worse in 1846 when his now ex-friend Morton organised an astounding demonstration of anaesthesia at Massachusetts General Hospital.

Morton and his associate Charles T. Jackson (1805–80) named their anaesthetic substance 'Letheon' and applied for a patent for it in October 1846, but everyone knew it was sulphuric ether, which, like nitrous oxide, was popular recreationally. Much bitterness ensued between Morton, Jackson and Wells as to who had employed anaesthesia first. Unknown to them at the time, it was someone else altogether. In 1849, Crawford Williamson Long (1815–78), a country doctor from Jackson County, Georgia, provided witness accounts that he had used ether in the removal of a tumour from the neck of James Venable on 30 March 1842.

Wells remained interested in anaesthetics but his mental health suffered. In 1848, under the influence of chloroform, he threw vitriol at two women and got arrested. He was allowed to go to his rooms to collect some possessions. Later, in the police cell, he anaesthetised himself before he razored open an artery in his thigh, taking his own life.

68. Chloroform Helped Her Majesty Give Birth

The chloroform that assisted Horace Wells' tragic death had been known in medicine since 1831, when Samuel Guthrie (1782–1848), a physician from Sackets Harbor, New York, produced it from chloride of lime and 'well-flavoured alcohol'. It was on the other side of the Atlantic, however, that its anaesthetic properties took off.

James Young Simpson (1811–70), an eminent Scottish obstetrician, was an enthusiastic proponent of ether and suspected other chemicals could have similar properties. On 4 November 1847, Simpson and his colleagues keeled over after testing chloroform and awoke with the realisation that it was good stuff. Chloroform was a quicker acting, better smelling anaesthetic, which required smaller doses than ether and was therefore more economical.

Just a few days later, Simpson administered it to Jane Carstairs, who was in labour with her second child. She was terrified and had not slept for days; her first labour had ended with the death of her baby son. Simpson later reported that she awoke from chloroform's refreshing slumber feeling better prepared for the task ahead of her, only to find that her daughter had already arrived. (The baby was named Wilhelmena, not Anaesthesia as legend would have it!)

A minority of people objected to chloroform on religious grounds, uneasy about the Bible's command that women would 'bring forth children in sorrow'. Simpson, himself a committed Christian, pre-empted criticism in his *Answer to the Religious Objections Advanced Against the Employment of Anaesthetic Agents in Midwifery and Surgery* (1847). Everyone loves a good science-versus-religion bunfight and the *Answer* sold well. As it happened, serious religious objectors were rare, but the self-promotion didn't do Simpson, or chloroform, any harm.

More pertinent were the medical objections. Concerns about chloroform's safety were justified; it was balancing people on the boundary of life and death. The first known chloroform fatality – fifteen-year-old Hannah Greener, who died during the removal of a severely ingrown toenail – was reported in January 1848, and increased the need for caution.

John Snow (1813–58) led the study of anaesthetic dosage, disagreeing with Simpson's early assertion that 'no special kind of inhaler or instrument is necessary'. Unlike the influential Simpson, Snow was an ordinary doctor, but from the moment of anaesthesia's introduction into Britain, he studied it with extraordinary dedication, and pioneered apparatus to administer it in a safe and scientific way.

On 7 April 1853, Snow administered chloroform to Queen Victoria during the birth of Prince Leopold. This must have been nerve-racking, as accidentally killing the Queen could have been slightly detrimental to his career. Fortunately, everything went to plan, and the event has been credited with silencing objections to anaesthesia. Snow, however, was discreet about Victoria's obstetrical history and the newspapers celebrated Leopold's arrival as the birth of a prince, not as the birth of a surgical innovation. In 1859, after Snow's death, several papers revealed that he had administered chloroform to the Queen six years earlier, apparently assuming this would be news to the public. By then, the non-royal populace had worked out for themselves that anaesthesia was brilliant.

69. Opium Had Its Teething Troubles

In Monroe, New York, in 1875, a tragic event hit the family of a seventeen-month-old boy. The child showed symptoms of worms and, by the advice of an acquaintance, his parents dosed him with fifteen to twenty drops of McMunn's Elixir of Opium every hour. The opium, they were told, would put the worms to sleep. Sadly, it also sent the baby to sleep ... for eternity. As the local newspaper poignantly put it: 'The little fellow was at play in the morning as ever and at eleven at night was a corpse.'

The use of opium in children's medicines was ubiquitous and controversial in America and Britain throughout the nineteenth century. Products such as Godfrey's Cordial and Mrs Winslow's Soothing Syrup promised to alleviate the pain of teething, leaving the little sufferer 'as bright as a button'. They were available without restriction from general stores and, along with chemists' own generic laudanum, were cheap enough for all strata of society.

Although critics of such products defined them as quackery, their status was ambiguous. McMunn's Elixir was prescribed by physicians; adverts in respectable medical journals promoted it as a safe, 'denarcotised' option. Teething coincided with the time of life where children were particularly vulnerable to disease, and parents may have felt that *not* using these pain-relieving products was too big a risk to take. The Pure Food and Drug Act of 1906 required the accurate labelling of opiate content but it was not until the 1920s that all sales of the drug were banned.

70. Semmelweis Encouraged Reluctant Doctors to Wash Their Hands

Let's say you've stumbled into a corner of the internet promoting a dodgy health supplement. Its miraculous cures, the website claims, have made doctors *furious*.

And then: bingo! The supplement-seller invokes Ignaz Semmelweis (1818–65), a Hungarian doctor famed for introducing disinfectant handwashing to the maternity wards of Vienna's general hospital in 1847.

As the usual story goes, Semmelweis noticed that childbed fever (post-partum sepsis) was more common after births assisted by doctors than those attended by midwives. He realised doctors were transmitting the disease by going straight to the ward from the autopsy table without washing their hands. His insistence on a good scrub was ridiculed by an egotistical medical profession; they soon put him in a madhouse and he died ... of sepsis.

It's a great morality tale. The message boils down to: 'They called Semmelweis mad, but he was right all along!', implying that our cure-seller is a persecuted visionary too.

Semmelweis did discover that 'cadaverous particles' from autopsies were causing the high death-rate; his introduction of hand disinfection with chloride of lime led to a dramatic reduction in mortality. The word 'disinfection' is key: far from being anathema, ordinary soap-and-water washing was already standard practice.

It is also true that Semmelweis's discoveries weren't welcomed with a big party. A clash of personalities with his boss, Johann Klein, brought some outspoken condemnation and an end to his employment. Others objected on scientific grounds. Carl Levy of Copenhagen maternity hospital pointed out how unlikely it was that a few particles on someone's fingers could be so deadly. Pasteur's work on germ theory would later show how infection spread, but in Semmelweis's time it was understandable to interpret the cadaverous matter as a poison, not a rapidly multiplying bacterium.

Semmelweis was not, however, universally scorned. Three influential medical figures, Ferdinand von Hebra, Josef Skoda and Karl von Rokitansky, supported his career ambitions and wrote and lectured about his ideas. Foreign obstetricians studying in Vienna also reported back to their own countries.

Semmelweis's discovery was preceded by the theory that childbed fever could pass from one patient to another (contagion). The difference with Semmelweis was his notion that decaying matter from *any* dead body or suppurating wound could cause infection. Not everyone grasped this distinction, as Semmelweis didn't publish his findings until 1861. When his *The Etiology, Concept and Prophylaxis of Childbed Fever* finally appeared, it included a rambling attack on his critics, which did not help him win people over.

In 1865, owing to what is now thought to be premature Alzheimer's disease, Semmelweis was taken to an asylum. In 1963, his remains were exhumed and historian Sherwin B. Nuland has since shown that his death resulted from violence by asylum staff, not sepsis. The truth, horrific enough in itself, lacks the poignant irony of the traditional version.

Semmelweis had a hard time, but his story can lend no legitimacy to the modern-day quacks who compare themselves with him. He should be remembered for saving countless lives, not used to validate people who think they're persecuted simply because their potion doesn't work.

71. NIGHTINGALE WAS GOOD AT NUMBERS AS WELL AS NURSING

The image of a statistician plotting a pie chart doesn't capture the public imagination quite as well as that of an angelic nurse gliding between rows of suffering war heroes, but Florence Nightingale's activities after the Crimean War saved more lives than anything she could do in the notorious Scutari Barrack Hospital.

Nightingale (1820–1910) arrived home from Scutari in August 1856 having witnessed thousands of preventable deaths. Of more than 21,000 British casualties, 16,323 had died of disease, not combat.

Soldiers who survived the crowded boat journey across the Black Sea to Scutari were dumped in an environment of filth and chaos, where bureaucratic ineptitude denied them medical supplies. Nightingale's organisation of sanitary improvements – ventilation, clean clothing and bedding, wound care, triage, nutrition, functional supply systems, etc. – had not immediately reduced the death rate. Deaths had risen over the winter of 1854 until she was able to get major works done on the faulty sewage system, after which mortality fell.

Nightingale lived with chronic illness during her post-Crimea years and, haunted by the 'frightful Scutari calamity', spent the rest of her life campaigning for sanitary reform. (The nature of her illness has been the subject of much discussion as to whether it involved mental health issues, the chronic effects of brucellosis or a psychosomatic attempt to get everyone to leave her alone so she could get on with her work. One thing is for sure – it wasn't syphilis, as a silly but persistent myth suggests.)

The nursing school at St Thomas's, her work to improve public health in India, the reform of workhouse nursing, the legacy of hospital infection control – all very interesting, but what about these scintillating pie charts?

Nightingale had always had an aptitude for mathematics, and amid the initial chaos of Scutari she established accurate record keeping. Her contributions to the Royal Sanitary Commission of 1857 included inventive ways of presenting this information to ensure it had an impact on politicians.

In her polar area diagram (she did not invent the format but pioneered its use as a tool for social change), the angle of each slice was equal but the radius was different according to the number being represented. This created a circle of wedges – each wedge showed the death rate for one month of the year, giving the numbers of soldiers who had died of preventable or mitigable diseases such as cholera and dysentery, those who had died of wounds, and deaths from other causes. The first section was huge, leaving the government in no doubt of the British Army's tragic failure to protect the health of its personnel. While the practical nursing skills for which Nightingale is popularly remembered undoubtedly made a difference to individual soldiers, it's the less romantic decades of organisational ability, pioneering epidemiology, and determination to influence those in power that became her lasting legacy.

72. Wine Helped Confirm Germ Theory

When Louis Pasteur (1822–95) was appointed dean of the science faculty at the University of Lille in 1854, ideas about microbes were already floating around the air like ... microbes. Friedrich Gustav Jakob Henle (1809–85) posited a germ theory of disease in his 1840 work *On Miasma and Contagia*. Expanding upon Fracastoro's notion of chemical 'seeds' of disease (see Fact 43), he suggested that the substance of contagion was organic and living. But it was still an abstract idea – no one had demonstrated what was really going on, and the bad air of miasma remained a popular explanation for disease.

Pasteur was a chemist, originally from Dole in France. At Lille, he began investigating alcohol fermentation problems in the local factories, finding that successful fermentations contained yeast cells, and the ones that had gone off contained bacteria as well. He researched fermentation over many years, later addressing the wine industry's difficulty with lactic acid turning the wine sour.

Sour wine, he found, was contaminated by microbes. Boiling it would kill them, but boiled wine is hardly a delectable accompaniment to one's coq au vin, so Pasteur experimented with heating it gently to about fifty degrees Celsius. This temperature destroyed the bacteria without rendering the wine completely rank. The process became known as pasteurisation and is now more commonly associated with dairy products. While working on fermentation, Pasteur also disproved the prevailing idea that microbes appeared by spontaneous generation. By using a new swan-neck container design, he enabled air to get to the contents while dust and bacteria got trapped – nothing could will itself into existence in these flasks.

This has to do with medicine because if microbes could

contaminate wine and beer and multiply therein, it was not unreasonable to suspect they could do the same in animals and humans. Pasteur and his wife Marie worked on diseases that were destroying France's silkworm industry, establishing that the silkworm eggs needed to be protected from airborne pathogens.

Pasteur continued to work on disease, studying anthrax and fowl cholera (which must have been nice for whichever heroic assistant got to clean out the chicken coop). While infecting some hens with cholera in 1879, he accidentally used an old, attenuated sample and conferred immunity on them. Pasteur began work on vaccines (a term he adopted in homage to Edward Jenner), developing them for rabies and anthrax in the 1880s.

The 1860–80s did not mark a sudden emergence out of the blue of some new-fangled thing called germ theory. It was something that had been brewing for centuries without a clear explanatory mechanism. Whereas Semmelweis had not been able to explain why tiny particles of decay could poison an adult human, Pasteur had the answer – microbes invaded the tissue and multiplied rapidly. Pasteur's work finally enabled a shift in the prevailing mindset so that germ theory could gain wide acceptance and act as the foundation for the development of effective new treatments.

73. THE FIRST AFRICAN AMERICAN WOMAN DOCTOR GRADUATED IN 1864

In May 1869, a doctor addressed the anniversary meeting of the New England Anti-Slavery Society. Slavery had been abolished in 1865, and the doctor expressed strong hopes for the future of the black race. She also gave a prescient warning: it would 'take earnest labour on the part of their friends to secure them all their rights'.

The speaker was Rebecca Crumpler who, at the height of the US Civil War, became the first African American woman to graduate as a physician. She devoted her career to improving the health status of black people living in poverty, especially women and children.

Born Rebecca Davis in Christiana, Delaware, in 1831, she spent her childhood in Pennsylvania with an aunt who acted as an informal healthcare practitioner and inspired her to enter a similar career. In 1852 she married Wyatt Lee and settled in Charlestown, Massachusetts. Until 1860, she worked as a nurse for local physicians then, with her employers' backing, was accepted into the New England Female Medical College. Her husband died of tuberculosis in 1863 but she persisted with her studies and graduated the following year as 'Doctress of Medicine.' She briefly practised in Boston before travelling to St John in New Brunswick, Canada, where she married Arthur Crumpler in May 1865.

With the Civil War now over, Crumpler went to Richmond, Virginia, to work for the Freedmen's Bureau, a government agency assisting freed slaves and poor whites in the former Confederate states. Despite her degree, she is listed in the bureau records as 'nurse', receiving $10 per month. As she explained in the introduction to her book, however, this part of her career was the 'real missionary work' to which she felt called. Serving a population of 30,000 black people emancipated from slavery yet still experiencing violent discrimination, she focused on assisting the poorest families.

A Book of Medical Discourses, one of the earliest medical publications by an African American writer, was based on Crumpler's journals and was specifically aimed at a female readership. She realised that knowledge is power and that encouraging women to be active in protecting their own and their children's health would improve their lives.

Although it's not clear to what extent Crumpler continued in medical practice towards the end of her life, she was still engaged in educating parents. In November 1891, in response to Boston's high infant mortality rate, Crumpler wrote to the *Boston Sunday Globe* emphasising that good nutrition and hygiene were more important than medicine.

She does not appear to have continued using the name 'Lee' after her second marriage, but is now remembered as Rebecca Lee Crumpler. Unfortunately there are no identified photographs of her. (Internet articles about her are often illustrated with a picture of Mary Eliza Mahoney, the first African American woman to graduate as a registered nurse.) Crumpler died in Boston in 1895 after an unostentatious life's work that put the needs of vulnerable people ahead of fame and fortune.

74. Antiseptics Made Surgery Safer

From 1861, two wards dealing with accidents and surgical cases at Glasgow Royal Infirmary belied the unsavoury image of the Victorian hospital. They were cleaned regularly, surfaces were disinfected with potassium permanganate; attendants washed their hands and dried them on spotless towels every time they changed a dressing. Yet wound infection remained a huge problem. The surgeon Joseph Lister (1827–1912), who had implemented these sanitary measures and made his wards a contrast to the less salubrious ones in the same building, needed to look further for a means of infection control.

Lister encountered Pasteur's ideas on fermentation in 1865. One accepted theory of wound infection held that the air's oxygen caused pus to form. Lister looked at infection from a different angle – what if the microorganisms responsible for fermentation also caused putrefaction in the flesh? If so, destroying these microorganisms before they got into the wound might prevent the usual terrible outcome.

Aware of the city of Carlisle's success at treating sewage with carbolic acid, Lister chose this substance as his antiseptic. In an 1867 paper in the *British Medical Journal* he explained that it 'appears to exercise a peculiarly destructive influence upon low forms of life' (sadly, the 1860s provided no opportunity for testing it on the comments sections of certain newspaper websites).

Lister started with compound fractures (where broken bones are accompanied by an open wound). The first goal was to destroy any germs by applying carbolic acid to every area of the wound (using a rag held in forceps). The next step aimed to guard against spreading decomposition by dressing the wound with a carbolic acid-soaked piece of lint, protected by a moulded tin cap that could be raised for the acid to be reapplied. For larger wounds, Lister introduced a paste of carbonate of lime, carbolic acid and boiled linseed oil, which he spread over a cloth dressing. Lister reported that in the first nine months of using these procedures, not a single case of hospital gangrene or pyaemia, once the scourge of the wards, had occurred.

His ideas provoked both criticism and praise. As with Semmelweis, some opposition arose due to misunderstandings about what the ideas actually were. James Young Simpson (the chloroform guy; also initially a critic of Semmelweis) highlighted various doctors who had used carbolic acid before, and grumpily argued that Lister was 'Not The First'. Another criticism arose from the assumption that carbolic acid was a miracle cure – some doctors splashed it about a bit and then blamed Lister when it didn't work.

The point, however, was the *antiseptic principle* – the defence of wounds against the microorganisms in the environment – not the stuff used to accomplish it. Lister frequently updated his techniques; in 1871, for example, he replaced carbolic acid with the alarming-sounding double cyanide of mercury and zinc, but the underlying principle remained the same. Enough surgeons adopted it with enthusiasm to bring it into general acceptance. It became possible to carry out operations that would previously have been precluded by the inevitability of infection.

75. THE EDINBURGH SEVEN CHALLENGED MISOGYNY IN MEDICINE

By 1869, women could take a medical degree at several universities in the United States and continental Europe, but not in Britain. Elizabeth Blackwell had received her degree in the US in 1849 and, when the Medical Register was established in 1858, her name was on it. Other women, however, could not follow, because the Register's rules changed to exclude anyone with a non-British degree.

Elizabeth Garrett (1836–1917) got onto the register by becoming a Licentiate of the Society of Apothecaries after receiving private tuition – but the Society then changed the rules to make private tuition unacceptable.

Sophia Jex-Blake (1840–1912) gained the conviction that medical education for women should be available in Britain too. Opponents claimed there was no demand for female doctors and that women did not have the strength for the medical life. Ironically, such opposition helped create the demand and forced Jex-Blake and her contemporaries to show just how tough they were.

The University of London would not admit her, so Jex-Blake tried Edinburgh, encouraging four other students to join her: Isabel Thorne, Edith Pechey, Matilda Chaplin and Helen Evans. They were admitted but had to pay higher fees and be taught separately from the men. A year later, Mary Anderson and Emily Bovell enrolled too, and the group became known as the Edinburgh Seven.

The women's presence at the university initially proved uneventful; this changed when their competence became clear. Edith Pechey's chemistry marks qualified her for the Hope Scholarship, which would give her free laboratory access. She was denied it because she had been taught separately from the official chemistry class, and the scholarship went to a man with lower marks.

In November 1870, the women went to Surgeons' Hall for an exam. A group of drunk male students slammed the gates in their faces. The women, however, did have support from other men on their course, and one of these let them in, facing the derision of his peers. The women completed their exam amid howls from outside, and the presence of a sheep, which the rioters had pushed into the hall. (The invigilator let it stay because it had more sense than the men outside.)

The women also experienced abuse in the streets and vitriol in the press. Their opponents' behaviour, however, backfired. The public started to wonder whether doctors condoning the shouting of obscenities at women could really be trusted with patients. Support for female doctors grew.

The University refused to award the Seven the degree of Doctor of Medicine, offering instead a meaningless 'certificate of proficiency'. In March 1874, when the women had exhausted all possibilities for medical education in Edinburgh, they moved on. Jex-Blake and Pechey took their degrees at Bern. Chaplin, Anderson and Bovell qualified at Paris; Thorne and Evans did not seek graduation but remained involved in women's medical education. Jex-Blake was instrumental in establishing medical schools for women in London and Edinburgh.

Spurred in part by the injustices faced by the Edinburgh Seven, the government passed a new Medical Act in 1876, legislating for the admission of women to the Medical Register.

76. Ugandan Surgeons Developed Life-Saving Caesarean Operations

Abdominal surgery to remove a child from the womb has a long history, but its purpose – and what constituted a success – changed over time. Although the operation's name is said to come from the birth of Julius Caesar, it's more likely to stem from the ancient Roman Law of the Caesars, which required it to be carried out when a woman died in childbirth. The procedure did not include any attempt to save the mother; it was about giving the child a chance of life or about separating the two individuals for purposes of burial. Occasional reports surfaced about operations resulting in a healthy mother and baby – in the year 1500, for example, a Swiss sow gelder called Jacob Nufer supposedly saved his wife and child in this way – but even after anaesthesia and antisepsis became available in the mid-to-late nineteenth century, a caesarean section remained a last resort for European and American surgeons.

In 1884, British doctors were therefore intrigued to learn that a sophisticated abdominal procedure had taken place five years earlier in the African kingdom of Bunyoro-Kitanga, whose inhabitants had experienced minimal contact with the rest of the world until the 1860s. In a lecture to the Edinburgh Obstetrical Society, medical missionary Robert W. Felkin (1853–1926) described a caesarean section carried out by Banyoro surgeons at Kahura, Uganda in 1879. Both mother and child had survived, and the expertise involved came as something of a surprise to those who saw Africans as a bunch of savages wandering about waiting for someone to come and civilise them.

The operation, Felkin reported, was carried out with

the intention of saving both lives. The mother, who was around twenty years old, was partially anaesthetised with banana wine. The surgeon also used this wine to wash the surgical site and his own hands, suggesting awareness of the need for infection control measures. He then made a vertical incision, going through the abdominal wall and part of the uterine wall, before further dividing the uterine wall enough to take the baby out. The operation also involved removing the placenta and squeezing the uterus to promote contraction.

The means of dressing the incision was also highly developed – the surgeon used seven polished iron spikes to bring the edges of the wound together, tying them in place with bark-cloth string. He then applied a thick layer of herbal paste and covered this with a warm banana leaf held in place with a bandage. According to Felkin's account, the mother and her baby were still doing well when he left the village eleven days later. Felkin took with him the knife used in the operation, and it is now part of the Wellcome Collection in London.

77. Certain Bacteria Caused Certain Diseases

Pasteur showed that microorganisms caused disease; Robert Koch (1843–1910) expanded upon this to develop ways of identifying *which* microorganism caused which disease.

His work on anthrax and cholera had precursors. Casimir Davaine found the anthrax bacillus in 1850 and later demonstrated that it had a role in the disease, although he did not discover its direct mode of transmission. Filippo Pacini studied the cadavers of cholera victims at the Santa Maria Nuova Hospital in Florence in 1854 and discovered 'vibrions', which he believed to cause the disease. He did not, however, try to grow a pure culture of it.

Koch improved the method of growing cultures of bacteria by using a solid rather than liquid medium – at first he grew them on raw potato but later developed agar plates. He was able to isolate the anthrax and cholera bacilli, linking specific microorganisms to specific diseases for the first time. With his colleague, Friedrich Loeffler (1852–1915), he set out 'Koch's postulates' – the four criteria that must be fulfilled to confirm that a bacterium caused a particular disease. The pathogen had to be abundant in every case of the disease, but not in healthy subjects; it had to be possible to isolate it from the diseased person or animal and grow it in a pure culture; this culture must then cause the disease in a healthy, susceptible laboratory animal; finally, the pathogen must be isolated again from the new host and shown to be identical to the original pathogen. These postulates applied principally to cholera and tuberculosis, and did not cover the viruses discovered in the 1890s. They have since been superseded by more detailed criteria.

In March 1882, Koch announced that he had identified the bacillus that caused tuberculosis, an event immediately recognised as momentous for the history of medicine. Ideas about miasma could be put back in the soil they'd seeped up from (although it did take a while for everyone to let go of them). So that was all great – we have a hero in the history of science.

But wait! Something strange then happened. Koch revealed in 1890 that he had developed a cure for tuberculosis. He claimed that the new substance, tuberculin, had prevented guinea pigs from contracting this fatal disease, and cured those already knocking on guinea pig heaven's door. Without adequate regulatory controls or quality standards, tuberculin was released amid much publicity to thousands of hopeful TB patients. It did not, however, work. Koch retained faith in tuberculin – a glycerin extract of the bacillus – and announced an improved version in 1897. It still didn't work, and the 'tuberculin scandal' damaged Koch's reputation.

The incongruity between Koch's contribution to the aetiology of tuberculosis and his subsequent failure with tuberculin reminds us that the human brain, no matter how clever and well-educated its individual owner, is susceptible to believing what it wants to believe. That's why scientific consensus is important – can the results of a study be replicated independently over and over again? The identification of pathogens could; the efficacy of tuberculin couldn't.

78. THE TAPEWORM MAN COULD GET RID OF YOUR UNWELCOME PASSENGERS

The beef tapeworm, *Taenia saginata*, can grow to over twenty metres long in the human intestines. It absorbs nutrients from the digestive system and can survive peacefully for years – unless, that is, its host attempts to evict it.

In early twentieth-century America, the tapeworm provided a profitable career for itinerant practitioners, who travelled from town to town parting people from their intestinal inhabitants. Such 'tapeworm specialists' are not exactly a celebrated part of the history of medicine, but their activities give an insight into the healthcare options available to rural communities.

Charles W. Oleson, in his 1890 book *Secret Nostrums and Systems of Medicine*, described how the worm doctor's treatment worked.

The patient must fast for a day, downing only a saline draught to empty the bowels. The next morning, he or she would take a teaspoon of the essential oil of male fern in a cup of warm milk. Milk was supposed to be 'an article of food in which the tapeworm greatly delights'. After this, the patient had to lie down for a few hours then have a dose of castor oil, turpentine and croton oil – the latter being toxic and a drastic laxative. The spectacular effects of this mixture can be imagined. Putting a piece of mosquito netting over your chamber pot meant 'the worm itself can be easily retained for further examination'.

The worm doctor is unlikely to be commemorated with a statue outside a hospital or a scholarly biography, but was part of the colourful variety of practitioners to whom the average person could turn when unable to afford a doctor.

79. The Snake Oil of the American West Was Really Made From Snakes ... Some of the Time

The phrase 'snake oil' – meaning something fraudulent and worthless – is now applied to a huge range of dodgy activities, from health gadgets to hollow political promises. The terminology originates from the late-nineteenth and early twentieth-century American showmen who promoted snake oil liniments through newspaper advertisements and dramatic exhibitions of snake handling. These products weren't always what they said on the tin. Such misleading snake oils, however, evolved from a more genuine traditional belief in the power of rattlesnake fat.

One oft-repeated snake oil origin story suggests that Chinese labourers on the First Transcontinental Railroad brought traditional water snake liniments to the US from 1864 onwards. In this narrative, the liniments' efficacy caught the attention of entrepreneurs, who substituted rattlesnakes for the water snakes and gradually dropped the snake content altogether.

This type of snake oil, used in Chinese medicine, was harvested from the fish-eating species *Enhydris chinensis*, which contains a high concentration of an omega-3 fatty acid with anti-inflammatory properties. There is, however, evidence that Americans were using home-grown rattlesnakes well before the arrival of the Chinese workers. It is from these earlier domestic remedies that the commercial snake oils evolved. (When people use the railroad labourers story to claim snake oil really worked, look out for whatever type of snake oil they're selling themselves.)

Native American tribes had long been aware of

the rattlesnake's potential – in 1762, French captain Jean-Bernard Bossu noted that the Choctaw used snake grease to ease rheumatic pains. This knowledge made its way into early nineteenth-century domestic medical books (an important resource for isolated pioneer families). While 'rattle-snake's oil' could also refer to a preparation of seneca (aka rattlesnake root), some sources make it clear they are talking about actual snakes.

Daniel J. Cobb's *The Family Adviser* (1828) listed rattlesnake oil alongside the oils of bear, hen, squirrel, goose, mud-turtle, skunk and wild cat, advising that it would 'soften a callus, and will thereby many times limber a stiff joint.' Five years later, *The Physician's Assistant* by Dr Brooks gave a variety of medicinal uses for rattlesnake. As well as using the oil internally or externally, one could take a teaspoon of powdered rattler flesh mixed in wine for 'all decays of the constitution'. Commercial rattlesnake oil was advertised at least as early as 1842 by druggists Clark and Collins in Montpelier, Vermont.

Later in the century, big-business patent medicine men turned snake oil into a shorthand for brash fakery. The best-remembered today is Clark Stanley's Snake Oil Liniment; other brands included Dr Clark's, George Atkins', Simm's, White Eagle and Miller's Antiseptic Oil, which carried the strapline 'known as Snake Oil'.

The 1906 Pure Food and Drug Act occasioned many prosecutions for misbranding. Clark Stanley's liniment was found in 1916 to consist of mineral oil, beef fat, capsicum and possible traces of camphor and turpentine.

The days of snake oil weren't over, as public demand remained high and genuine rattlesnake products were still being made. It had become associated, however, with the showmanship, wild claims and misrepresentation that characterise the metaphorical 'snake oil' in today's usage.

80. A Hospital Romance Brought Rubber Gloves into the Operating Theatre

During the winter of 1889/90 Caroline Hampton, chief nurse of the operating theatre at Johns Hopkins University Hospital, developed contact dermatitis from disinfectants.

Because she was 'an unusually efficient woman', the surgery department chief, William Stewart Halsted, asked the Goodyear Rubber Company to make her two pairs of thin latex gloves. A few months after this romantic gesture, Halsted and Hampton got married and were together for thirty-two years, dying two months apart in 1922.

Although Halsted was a keen proponent of infection control, it did not immediately occur to him that the gloves could be part of this. It was his chief assistant surgeon, Joseph 'Bloody' Bloodgood who (apart from having the best name out of everybody) was the first to realise the gloves' potential for preventing infection.

In 1896, Bloodgood began insisting that all members of the surgical team use latex gloves, and in 1899 he reported the resulting improvement in rates of infection in inguinal hernia operations.

Attempts to kill bacteria were already rigorous – operating theatre staff routinely scrubbed their hands with green soap and very hot water, then used potassium permanganate and oxalic acid before soaking their hands and forearms in 1:1,000 solution of bichloride for at least five minutes. But even this wasn't enough to stop 9.6 per cent of a sample of 104 hernia patients from getting suppurating wounds. After Bloodgood ensured operators as well as assistants wore gloves sterilised by boiling and bichloride, only 1.7 per cent of a further 226 hernia sites got infected. The difference in infection rates was self-evident and gloves became widely adopted.

81. PLAGUE RETURNED (THOUGH IT NEVER REALLY WENT AWAY)

Plague. Such a short word, and yet one so evocative of both physical agony and widespread social breakdown. Disorder and disease turn everything upside down. After the plague, nothing can ever be the same again.

The Third Plague Pandemic finished within living memory, yet is little known in Europe – probably because it happened to 'them' instead of 'us'. Previous pandemics had wiped people out indiscriminately. This one disproportionately affected those living in poverty, highlighting the global health inequality that has been worsening ever since.

The Third Plague Pandemic emerged in China in the 1850s and crossed international borders during the 1890s. (Pandemics one and two were the Plague of Justinian in 541–2 CE and the Black Death. There could have been earlier ones as well, but dividing them into three is the current convenient way of referring to them.) From Hong Kong in 1894, rats infested with plague-carrying fleas starting travelling the world on colonial supply ships, taking their lethal bacteria to every inhabited continent. They reached India in 1896, Egypt in 1899, the United States, Australia and Scotland in 1900, the West Indies and South America in 1908.

The bacterium responsible for bubonic plague was isolated in 1894 by Alexandre Yersin and Kitasato Shibasaburō, who independently discovered it within days of each other. Yersin found it in both rodents and humans, suggesting a connection, and in 1898 Paul-Louis Simond established rat fleas as the vector. As the disease spread to international ports, public health officials responded with quarantine programmes that isolated suspected sufferers and their families on the assumption that the disease could pass from one human to another.

Draconian measures by the British government in India led to political unrest; in the United States, existing anti-Asian prejudice fed on the disease's Chinese origin. When plague reached Cape Town via Argentina in 1901, its first victims were black dock workers. South Africa's colonial government used this as a pretext to remove the African population of District Six, forcing them under armed guard to a location outside the city at Uitvlugt (Ndabeni). Segregation, which had been regularly mooted on ostensible health grounds for the previous two decades, began in earnest.

The Third Pandemic killed around fifteen million people, the majority in India and Africa. Although the disease's pandemic status officially ended in 1959, plague has never been eradicated. Madagascar is the current most severely affected country – the World Health Organisation reported 263 cases there between September 2014 and February 2015. Seventy-one people died.

Reliable diagnostic tests can catch plague early and the bacterium *Yersinia pestis* remains susceptible to the same antibiotics that treated it in the 1940s and 50s – streptomycin is the first-line drug. Yet to say 'it's OK folks, we have antibiotics now!' feels a bit like being the bloke in an old war movie who shows his buddy a picture of his family. In the 1990s, multi-drug resistant strains of *Y. pestis* appeared in Madagascar, and the insecticide deltamethrin is no longer always effective against fleas. Will future historians find themselves analysing the Fourth Plague Pandemic?

82. X-RAYS REVEALED THE BODY'S SECRETS

The German physicist Wilhelm Röntgen (1845–1923) deserves much credit for keeping his cool in the face of extraordinarily creepy goings-on. Near midnight on 8 November 1895, he was experimenting with a cathode ray tube in a dark room when an ethereal glow appeared on the nearby barium platinocyanide-coated card. Objects placed in between the cathode ray tube and the card did not block whatever was causing this phenomenon.

It was like all that weird ectoplasm stuff that spiritualists kept claiming to find. But this was definitely real. Röntgen continued to investigate by placing different materials in the way. Then, as his fingers passed in front of the card, he saw it – a skeletal hand. *An animated skeletal hand*. Thanks to him having the presence of mind not to burn the house down and run screaming from the universe, the unknown rays causing the effect would become a major diagnostic tool.

The uroscopy of the medieval era and the stethoscope of 1816 shared a goal – to reveal what was going on inside the body and to create a window to its mysteries. Now, the window was beginning to open.

Röntgen's paper *Eine Neue Arte von Strahlen* (*A New Kind of Rays*), was published in December 1895, coining the term 'X-rays' for this unknown quantity. He also had it printed privately and sent it to a few scientific colleagues, accompanied by a photographic print that would become one of the most famous images in the history of science – the bones of his wife Bertha Röntgen's left hand, showing her wedding ring. This astounding picture captured the imagination of the public as well as the scientific world. Newspapers publicised the 'photography of the invisible' and its Gothic power to reveal to the observer his or her own 'death's head'.

Röntgen had no medical applications in mind when making his experiments, but the X-rays' diagnostic potential was immediately obvious to surgeons, and in January 1896 British surgeon John Hall-Edwards (1858–1926) used X-rays to reveal the whereabouts of a needle stuck in a patient's hand; the photograph was used as a guide for surgeons to remove it. A few weeks later, Hall-Edwards also located a bullet lodged in a boy's hand and was able to make an informed decision to leave it where it was.

During 1896, the therapeutic potential of X-rays gained widespread attention. Researchers working with them experienced skin burns reminiscent of the caustic salves used to treat growths and easily accessible cancers. X-rays became particularly useful in the treatment of basal cell carcinoma.

The new science, however, wasn't all serious. In summer 1896, London's Royal Aquarium offered a novel attraction: 'See your bones with the X-rays!' A gossip columnist in the *Exeter Flying Post* facetiously predicted that twentieth-century people would adorn their homes with portraits of their skeletons, and those not outwardly blessed with good looks would find their aesthetic niche in 'bone beauty competitions'. Most importantly, the *New York Tribune* reported, X-rays showed potential to be used in theatres by 'the unhappy victim of the big hat.'

83. RADIUM BROUGHT HOPE TO CANCER PATIENTS

Like Röntgen, Marie Curie did not expect her research to end up in hospital. In May 1896, just a few months after Röntgen's announcement of X-rays, Henri Becquerel (1852–1908) discovered that uranium emitted a similar type of ray of its own accord. To the public, still revelling in the excitement of seeing their own bones, Becquerel's rays weren't much of a novelty. Rays had been done. They were, however, of great interest to Marie Skłodowska Curie (1867–1934), who was looking for a research project for her PhD.

Curie was a Polish physicist working at the Sorbonne in Paris, and investigated the uranium rays by measuring the conductivity of the air they passed through. She tested all other known elements and found that only one – thorium – exhibited similar properties. Curie called the phenomenon 'radioactivity' and theorised that it was an atomic property of the elements that remained constant regardless of light, temperature and the element's chemical state.

She found that an ore of uranium called pitchblende was far more radioactive than uranium itself, suggesting that unknown radioactive elements were in there somewhere. Curie's husband Pierre joined the project and in 1898, after much arduous work, they succeeded in isolating two previously unknown elements, which they named polonium and radium. The amounts were tiny – it took a ton of pitchblende to get two or three decigrams of radium.

Radium, like X-rays, caused skin lesions, and in 1899/1900 dentist Friedrich Walkoff and chemist Friedrich Giesel in Germany conducted tests on their own skin – an experiment subsequently tried by Becquerel and the Curies too. X-rays were already in use therapeutically and it was a short step for doctors to start trying radioactivity in the cure of certain conditions. Henri-Alexandre Danlos and Eugène Bloch successfully treated lupus vulgaris – a tubercular skin disease – in 1901, using radium supplied by the Curies.

Radium being expensive and difficult to get hold of, interested doctors had to beg or borrow some from acquaintances, and clinical use was patchy until 1903, when S. W. Goldberg and Efim London in St Petersburg announced the successful treatment of basal cell carcinoma (also known as a rodent ulcer). By this time, commercial factories (including one run by Friedrich Giesel) were producing radium in sufficient quantities for its use to become widespread. (Quantities that were still minuscule, but once a hospital had some, they could use it again and again.)

The usual early format of treatment was a radium salt such as radium bromide in small glass tubes. In the case of basal cell carcinoma and similarly accessible diseases, the tubes could be attached directly over the growth with adhesive strips. As the number of cancers that responded to radium therapy increased, so did the ingenious instruments and moulds designed to target the radioactivity directly at the tumour.

There was (and remains) much work still to do on the treatment of cancers, and radium also had its dangerous side, but the Curies' commitment to science for its own sake provided a medical breakthrough upon which later generations of researchers could build.

84. Quackbusters Tried to Crack Down on Medical Fraud ...

'Quackery' can be hard to define, but essentially refers to misleading claims for health products or services of questionable validity, advertised for financial gain. In the early twentieth century, medical campaigners attempted to educate the public about the methods employed by unscrupulous practitioners.

In the US, mail-order schemes selling worthless or damaging remedies were a multi-million-dollar industry, and fraudulent businesses used high-pressure sales techniques to woo their customers. One such product was Habitina, which claimed to cure drug addiction. Advertisements attracted addicts' attention with the large heading 'MORPHINE' – and that's exactly what was in the bottle. By using Habitina, the purchaser could get a fix of narcotics while telling their family they were under treatment.

Some companies offered free samples in order to harvest names and addresses, which they then bombarded with junk mail. The Magic Foot Draft Company offered a big sticky plaster supposed to draw impurities out through the soles of the feet. The business, like many others, was relentless in the volume of correspondence it sent to prospective customers, badgering them to buy the products.

Samuel Hopkins Adams (1871–1958) was a journalist who put his talent for muckraking to work against scandals in public health provision and medical fraud. In 1905, *Collier's National Weekly* commissioned him to write a series of articles on patent remedies, and these were published as *The Great American Fraud*. In them, he named and shamed more than 260 popular medicines.

Adams knew vendors would respond with a 'Not All

Quacks Are Like That' argument, claiming it was unfair to lump proprietary medicines together as a bad thing. He didn't buy this at all. 'This honest attempt', he wrote, 'to separate the sheep from the goats develops a lamentable lack of candidates for the sheepfold'.

Adams wasn't the only one writing about health issues, and the heightened public awareness created the environment for the passage of the Pure Food and Drug Act in 1906. This didn't ban patent medicines but obliged manufacturers to label them with the ingredients and refrain from making misleading claims. It did not, however, cover medical devices, which soon proliferated.

At about this time, the American Medical Association's Propaganda Department (later the less sinister-sounding Bureau of Investigation) was joined by Arthur J. Cramp, who devoted his career to educating the public about quackery. He published pamphlets exposing the reality of such products as 'Obesity Cures' and 'Cancer Cures', later compiling these into three books under the title *Nostrums and Quackery* between 1911 and 1936.

The secrecy surrounding the remedies' ingredients also concerned the British Medical Association, which started printing analyses in its journal in 1908, publishing them as books called *Secret Remedies* and *More Secret Remedies* in 1909 and 1912. They revealed what the medicines contained and the mark-up on the cost of ingredients. In time-honoured fashion, both American and British campaigners received accusations of professional jealousy, arrogance and incompetence from those whose businesses they targeted.

Did they succeed in ridding society of unscientific remedies and practitioners prepared to peddle false hope? A hundred years later, any time spent on the Internet quickly reveals that they didn't.

85. ... BUT THAT DIDN'T INCLUDE TAPEWORM DIET PILLS

In these days of wacky weight-loss schemes and 'one weird tip' discoveries featuring an ordinary mum who has incurred the wrath of the medical profession for some unspecified reason, the tapeworm diet has once again wriggled its way into the public consciousness. Occasional reports surface of someone ingesting tapeworm eggs in order to shed the pounds, and such drastic measures claim a long historical pedigree. Victorian women, says the Internet, took tapeworm pills in order to keep their figures slender.

There is, however, very little evidence that tapeworms ever found their way into commercial weight loss products. The legend appears to have started in the US in 1912, when a news dispatch from Peoria, Illinois, claimed that a society woman had ordered a miracle diet pill only for her husband to send it to Washington for analysis and discover that it contained the head of a tapeworm. When asked, however, the Washington analysts had never heard of such a story; Surgeon General Rupert Blue (1868–1948) wrote it off as a 'fine yarn'.

Over the next fifty years, the American Medical Association received numerous enquiries from concerned members of the public, who had heard that diet products could contain more than anyone bargained for. Newspapers, too, relished the chance to resurrect the story at regular intervals. In 1953, a newspaper agony uncle called Dr Edwin P. Jordan received a letter from a fellow physician claiming that three of his patients had bought pills whose packaging stated: 'Contains the ova of taenis [sic] saginata.' Unfortunately, the AMA's efforts to pin down the details met with a dead end.

The early twentieth-century versions of the tale cast the tapeworm in the role of imposter – unsuspecting dieters bought pills in good faith and were horrified to find out what they really were. One fictional account appeared in Mabel Herbert Urner's popular newspaper column, *The Married Life of Helen and Warren*, in 1927. The character of Mrs Dodson, who buys some suspicious-looking slippery grey capsules from Dr Phake, fits the bill to become everyone's grandma's 'friend of a friend' who left her pills in a warm place and returned to find them wriggling.

As reports surfaced in the 1950s that the opera singer Maria Callas had deliberately undergone tapeworm infestation under medical supervision, the story evolved to include people who teamed up with tapeworms on purpose out of vanity. (Callas did suffer from them, but probably got them in the usual way through her diet.)

Modern representations of historical wormy tablets include a famous advertisement for 'Sanitized Tape Worms' – it promises that you can 'Eat! Eat! Eat! & Always Stay Thin!' Much of its artwork, however, is lifted from 1920s advertisements for another weight-loss product called Neutroids, which contained iodol, magnesium carbonate, starch, talc and a trace of iron – but no tapeworms. As a vintage-inspired joke poster, Sanitized Tape Worms are just a bit of fun, and carry on a legend that most likely wormed its way out of a journalist's imagination.

86. Insulin Transformed the Outlook for People with Diabetes

Diabetes is an ancient condition. Even the name 'diabetes' dates back to the Ancient Greeks, and the disease itself was known to the Egyptians in the second millennium BCE. What is now called Type 1 diabetes is an auto-immune disease that destroys the cells producing the hormone insulin. Without insulin, glucose can't get into the rest of the body's cells and they have to find fuel from elsewhere, breaking down tissue and releasing by-products that can ultimately lead to coma and death.

Many treatments, including dietary ones, had been tried over the centuries; on the eve of insulin's availability, the method in vogue was led by Frederick M. Allen (1879–1964). The 'Allen Plan' severely reduced patients' calorie intake until they weren't excreting glucose in their urine. It then built up to a low but survivable calorie level tailored to the individual. The treatment was grim for the patient and offered minimal increases in longevity. In 1915, when it became established, there were few other options; that, however, was soon to change.

From 1889, when Oscar Minkowski and Josef von Mering showed that removal of the pancreas induced diabetes in dogs, scientists knew that a pancreatic secretion must be controlling blood glucose.

Lydia De Witt in 1906 isolated the islets of Langerhans from cats, suggesting that they were the origin of the secretion. The same year, George Zülzer tested a pancreatic extract he called 'Acomatrol' on patients, but its side effects outweighed the benefits. In 1909, Jean De Meyer suggested the term 'insuline' (from the Latin word for 'island'). Between 1915 and 1919, Israel Kleiner proved conclusively that pancreatic material regulated blood sugar levels.

One of the most controversial figures in insulin's history is the Romanian physiologist Nicolae Paulescu (1869–1931). He extracted a substance he called 'pancréine' – now recognised as insulin – in 1916, but had to postpone his work during the war and could not publish it until 1921. By then, he had not yet purified the extract to an extent that would make it usable in humans. Paulescu's scientific achievements have since held a low profile owing to his abhorrent opinions about Jews and his involvement in the fascist politics of the time.

Frederick Banting (1891–1941), working under the auspices of Professor John J. R. Macleod (1876–1935) at Toronto University, began experimenting on dogs in 1921. He and his assistant, Charles Best (1899–1978) succeeded in obtaining an extract that perked up pancreas-less pooches. By January 1922, they were ready to test it on a human patient – fourteen-year-old Leonard Thompson, who was on the verge of a diabetic coma.

Thompson had an allergic reaction and Macleod brought in biochemist James Bertram Collip (1892–1965), who refined the extract and made it safer for clinical use. Thompson's second injection rapidly improved his condition and he survived by using insulin for thirteen years. Banting and Macleod received the Nobel Prize in Physiology or Medicine in 1923. Banting shared his prize money with Best, and Macleod shared his with Collip, which all sounds like a happy-tears group-hug moment, but was actually fraught with passive aggression and egotism.

Still, the end result was that people with diabetes could live a normal life, so that's the main thing.

87. The Army Battled Against the Common Cold

The trouble with having a cold is that you can feel as though you're about to drop dead in a festering pile of slimy tissues, and yet no one takes you seriously. The duties of life must go on; work must be done and children fed even when your head is a cauldron of snot soup. No wonder people try to dignify their suffering with the grander appellation of 'flu'.

In the 1920s, however, the US Chemical Warfare Service decided to give the common cold the fight it deserved. Their methods contributed to a brief trend among physicians for chlorine therapy – one of those episodes in the history of medicine that is now largely forgotten but that could have been momentous ... if it had worked.

During the influenza pandemic of 1918–19, the hospitals at the CWS's Edgewood Arsenal, Maryland, were overflowing. Doctors observed an interesting phenomenon – workers from the chlorine gas plant were not among those suffering. Could chlorine prevent the further spread of the Spanish flu? Preliminary experiments at the University of Arkansas produced encouraging but inconclusive results. In 1922, the CWS chief General Amos Alfred Fries (1873–1963), who was fighting to keep the service operational in the face of public and military opposition to chemical warfare, saw the chance for a great public relations coup. He appointed Colonel Edward Bright Vedder (1878–1952, now better remembered for his work on beriberi) to head up further investigations.

Vedder and his colleague, Captain Harold P. Sawyer, focused on colds rather than flu. Sniffling volunteers sat in an enclosed chamber for one hour, breathing in a concentration of 0.015 micrograms of chlorine per litre of air.

In a paper published in March 1924, Vedder and Sawyer reported that 71.4 per cent of their patients were 'cured' and 23.4 per cent 'improved'. This they attributed to chlorine's bactericidal action, to increased production of mucus to flush pathogens away, and to migration of white blood cells to where they were needed.

Vedder, a conscientious scientist, was circumspect about his results, but the CWS needed a big announcement about its efforts for the good of humanity. When Fries arranged for President Calvin Coolidge to have chlorine treatment for a cold, the story was a hit with the newspapers and the public. Chlorine chambers became the first resort in the battle against bunged-up noses.

The treatment also came under criticism. The New York Board of Health pointed out that most colds got better anyway. Randomised, double-blind, placebo-controlled trials were not yet the norm, so Vedder had not used a control group. Further experiments at the University of Minnesota showed that most people recovered within a week regardless of whether they had chlorine, other medications or nothing at all.

The chlorine treatment faded away as quickly as it had emerged, partly because the Chemical Warfare Service had moved on to other things – the development of insecticides was a more profitable peacetime use for its resources. Humanity's thousands of years of sneezing continued unabated.

88. THE FRONTIER NURSING SERVICE TOOK PRIMARY CARE TO RURAL COMMUNITIES

All the medical developments in the world are no use if you can't access them. In early twentieth century Kentucky, the isolated mountain communities had not one licensed physician to turn to. In response to their situation, a complex public health pioneer introduced a team of nurses who didn't let mountains, forests or rivers get in their way.

Mary Breckinridge (1881–1965) opened the Frontier Nursing Service in 1925, employing nurse-midwives trained in Britain. Beginning with a clinic at Hyden, it grew to six outposts, each serving around 250 families, and a purpose-built twelve-bed hospital. The nurses travelled on horseback to the remote homes, carrying their equipment in saddlebags. Fording swollen rivers, dodging quicksand and negotiating narrow mountain trails were all in a day's work.

The image of dedicated nurses battling through the wilderness provided the perfect fundraising tool, and Breckinridge was adept at gaining support from the wealthy social circles into which she had been born. Breckinridge also recognised the fundraising importance of statistics – she was able to prove a demonstrable reduction in infant and maternal mortality that encouraged donors' generosity.

Support for the FNS, however, also arose from what can now be recognised as a more sinister motivation. Breckinridge presented the Appalachian people as the finest, purest white American stock, whose preservation was essential in the face of perceived racial degeneration. This conflict between Breckinridge's undoubted commitment to child welfare and her views on race reflect a common occurrence in the history of medicine – people superficially characterised as heroes or villains were complicated individuals operating within the social and political context of their time.

89. PENICILLIN DRIFTED IN BY CHANCE ...

The idea of using mould for healing dated (like most things) back to Ancient Egypt, but as studies of bacteria increased in the late nineteenth century, the germ-killing properties of moulds – especially *Penicillium* species – sporadically cropped up. (Or should that be *spore-adically*? Ha!)

In 1871, for example, Joseph Lister used *Penicillium glaucum* to treat a nurse's infected injury, and four years later physicist John Tyndall (1820–93) found that his experiments into the distribution of airborne bacteria had been contaminated by a *Penicillium* mould that was bumping off his germs. Yet this was before Robert Koch's work in identifying specific pathogens, so the full medical potential of this accident wasn't obvious. Then in 1897, a medical student called Ernest Duchesne (1874–1912) in Lyons investigated the action of *P. glaucum* for his dissertation. His experiments on typhoid-infected guinea pigs had encouraging results, but Duchesne never got the opportunity to expand upon his findings. From 1915 through the 1920s, Costa Rican scientist Clodomiro Picado Twight (1887–1944) also carried out experiments to assess the antibacterial effects of penicillium.

These encounters with penicillium (and there were others too) showed antibiosis – where one microorganism destroys another – but they did not result in a therapeutically viable drug. That process began with the observational acuity of Scottish bacteriologist Alexander Fleming (1881–1955), working at St Mary's Hospital in London.

It's one of the best-known moments in the history of medicine. In September 1928, Fleming returned from holiday to discover a fluffy mould on a neglected agar plate of *Staphylococcus aureus*. Later retellings credited an open window with allowing this wandering spore to float romantically into the future of the human race. Penicillium moulds were under study elsewhere in the same building, however, so there were a lot of them about. Fleming noticed that the mould had a 'halo' of transparent staphylococci. Something exuding from this mould – which he at first thought was *P. rubrum* but later turned out to be a potent variant strain of *P. notatum* – was destroying the bacterial membranes.

In his 1929 paper, *On the Antibacterial Action of Cultures of a Penicillium, with Special Reference to their Use in the Isolation of B. influenzae*, Fleming noted that he had made a broth culture filtrate of the mould. This he named 'penicillin', to avoid having to use the cumbersome phrase 'mould broth filtrate' all the time. Even large doses had proved non-toxic in lab animals, and Fleming suggested the filtrate had potential for antisepsis in wounds and for isolating non-susceptible bacteria for study (i.e. if you had a sample containing several bacteria species, you could wipe out most of them and keep the one you wanted).

Fleming did not, however, test penicillin as an internally administered drug, perhaps because the general scientific climate was pessimistic about finding antimicrobial substances safe and effective enough for use. Over the next decade, penicillin mainly survived as a laboratory tool – but the Second World War precipitated a fresh look at Fleming's findings and a huge transatlantic effort to produce penicillin in life-saving quantities.

90. ... But It Took a Lot of People to Make a Lot of It

For penicillin to be of use to society, there needed to be lots of it. Loads and loads. In 1939, Oxford-based Australian pathologist Howard Florey (1898–1968) and his colleague Ernst Chain (1906–79), a biochemist who had escaped Nazi Germany, revisited Fleming's work with a view to producing penicillin on a large scale.

By this time, sulphonamide antibacterial drugs – principally Prontosil developed by Gerhard Domagk in Germany from red azo dye – were on the market. This changed things; it was clear that antibacterials taken internally could cure infection. Florey's team experimented with penicillin on mice injected with fatal doses of streptococcus. Those who received penicillin survived much longer than their luckless control-group friends.

The spores that had contaminated Alexander Fleming's Petri dish weren't just any old mould but a variant strain that yielded more penicillin than bog-standard *P. notatum*. (This is central to why Fleming is credited for the discovery of penicillin rather than the other scientists whose penicillium investigations pre-dated his.) This strain was what was Florey's team used, yet penicillin remained unstable and difficult to produce in quantity; gallons of mould broth would yield only a small amount of the 'juice'. Nevertheless, the team went into production, using porcelain vessels designed by Norman Heatley (1911–2004) to grow the mould.

Florey stressed that the development of penicillin was a team effort. When the results appeared in the *Lancet* in 1940, seven people were listed as co-authors – Chain, Florey, Arthur D. Gardner, Norman Heatley, Margaret

Jennings, Jean Orr-Ewing, and Gordon Sanders. All had made essential individual contributions to the work, supported by lab technicians and the six 'Penicillin girls' employed to do the legwork in the 'factory' that had sprung up in Florey's lab.

After the *Lancet* paper came out, scientists in the US joined in the efforts to develop a therapeutic-quality drug. At Columbia University, Henry Dawson, Gladys L. Hobby and Karl Meyer produced penicillin from a Fleming mould sample, and carried out the first human trials in December 1940.

With war draining British resources, Florey found the drug companies reluctant to take on mass production of penicillin so in the summer of 1941 he and Norman Heatley travelled to the US to drum up interest there. The US Northern Regional Research Center in Peoria, Illinois, took up the cause of searching for penicillium strains that would yield lots of penicillin. In 1943, Dorothy I. Fennell isolated just such a strain from a mouldy cantaloupe from the local market. Elizabeth McCoy of the University of Wisconsin went on to engineer a mutant strain that yielded 900 times as much penicillin as Fleming's original. Commercial production became possible, enabling the use of penicillin for injured soldiers during the war and, afterwards, for civilians too.

Fleming, Florey and Chain shared the Nobel Prize for Medicine in 1945, becoming figureheads for a process of development involving thousands of contributions. The same year, Dorothy Hodgkin used X-ray crystallography to confirm the chemical construction of the penicillin molecule, opening the opportunity for the production of synthetic penicillin-like drugs.

91. TWENTIETH-CENTURY CONDITIONS WERE RIPE FOR POLIO OUTBREAKS

Poliovirus was the ninja of pathogens. For millennia, it thrived everywhere, unseen by its human hosts. Poliovirus sailed through digestive systems in silence, emerging into nappies and privies unheeded, contaminating water supplies, nestling under fingernails. Just occasionally, it made a foray into a child's central nervous system, causing paralysis – perhaps even death – before retreating once more into the unknown.

Then, in late nineteenth-century Europe and America, poliovirus rushed out of hiding. Children were out playing in the morning and irreversibly paralysed by bedtime. By 1916, the disease – at first called infantile paralysis and later poliomyelitis – had reached epidemic proportions in the US and would return every summer.

About 90 per cent of poliovirus infections are subclinical. Most of those who do get symptoms experience temporary fever and stiffness resulting from the virus entering the bloodstream. Just one in two hundred poliovirus infections causes paralysis by destroying neurones – so a single severe case of polio in the community indicates that the virus is already at epidemic levels.

The probable cause of the early twentieth-century outbreaks now seems counter-intuitive. Improvements in sanitation and awareness of germs had inadvertently prevented very young babies from getting the asymptomatic poliovirus infections that had affected the generations before them. Most would encounter the virus eventually, but not until they were older, when it was more likely to result in disability.

In 1927, Philip Drinker and Louis Agassiz Shaw invented an artificial respirator that became known as the iron lung. By using alternate negative and positive pressures to make the chest rise and fall, it kept people alive in the acute first stages of the disease where chest muscles became paralysed. Jack Emerson created a lighter, cheaper design that became a familiar feature of hospitals. For a minority of polio survivors with permanent respiratory paralysis, the iron lung became home, keeping them breathing for the rest of their lives – sometimes for as much as sixty years.

In the 1930s, Australian nurse Elizabeth Kenny introduced a system of physical therapy that used heat packs and exercises to improve mobility. Her system ran contrary to the common practice of using splints to keep limbs still, and she encountered opposition – not least because she was self-taught as a nurse and didn't have any official qualifications. Her methods, however, had gained acceptance by the 1940s.

Despite the importance of assisting people who already had the disease, scientific research focused on preventing the annual outbreaks from recurring. In 1955, the announcement of Jonas Salk's (1914–95) vaccine using 'killed' poliovirus resulted in countrywide celebrations. The end of this devastating disease seemed to be nigh, and within a decade, cases in the US had plummeted to the hundreds rather than the thousands. An orally administered live vaccine created by Albert Sabin (1906–93) became available in 1961, becoming the preferred choice for mass immunisation campaigns, where it could be administered by volunteers without medical training. Both vaccines have helped bring the worldwide eradication of poliovirus within our grasp.

92. THE US PUBLIC HEALTH SERVICE CARRIED OUT AN INFAMOUSLY UNETHICAL STUDY

In 1972, investigative journalist Jean Heller exposed a shocking episode in American medical history. Whistleblowers from within the US Public Health Service revealed that for forty years the service had been observing the course of syphilis among African American men – and denying them treatment.

The 'Tuskegee Study of Untreated Syphilis in the Negro Male' began as a six-month observational study in 1932. Macon County, Alabama, was identified as an area of prevalent syphilis, and to recruit people for the study, the USPHS promoted a 'free healthcare' programme. Tests identified 399 men with syphilis in a latent, asymptomatic stage. Those accepted onto the programme were diagnosed with 'bad blood' and told that the medicines they were given (mostly aspirin, but initially inadequate doses of syphilis medication too) constituted treatment.

This was before penicillin, but the arsenic-based drug neosalvarsan was available. With the Great Depression under way and no funding for this drug, the USPHS extended the study to observe the disease's natural course until the men's deaths. Just over 200 men without syphilis were recruited in 1933 as a control group.

From 1945, penicillin was the main treatment for syphilis and in 1947, the Nuremberg Code established ethical principles of human medical research in the aftermath of the Nazi war crimes. The Code asserted that: *The voluntary consent of the human subject is absolutely essential.*

Neither of these developments changed the Tuskegee study. The men were not offered penicillin and still did not have the accurate information required to give consent.

A persistent myth circulates that the study involved the purposeful injection of the men with syphilis bacteria. This is not true; they already had the disease. The withholding of treatment, however, did lead to people becoming infected during the study – particularly their wives and children. At least forty women contracted syphilis and nineteen babies were born with it.

Although John R. Heller (former director of the PHS venereal disease section) was quoted in 1972 as saying 'There was no racial side to this. It just happened to be in a black community', there is now no doubt that the study was embedded in racist stereotypes about black men's sexuality and their relationship with healthcare.

Syphilis, these attitudes implied, had not been a problem during the era of slavery, but freedom had enabled black people to revert to immorality. Syphilis was considered such a 'natural' part of black men's lives that they wouldn't bother to seek treatment. If they weren't going to be treated anyway, the course of their disease might as well be observed.

In 2004, the last surviving participant, Ernest Hendon, died at the age of ninety-six. Just a few years previously, he attended a ceremony at Alabama's House of Representatives, where the state expressed its regret for its role in the study.

'Everybody knows now that we were mistreated,' Hendon reportedly said. 'I'm glad they're seeing now that it will never happen again.' But for many, the legacy of Tuskegee is the fear that it *could* happen again. Institutional racism is far from eradicated, and Tuskegee remains a symbol for centuries of injustice against black people.

93. THE PIONEER OF BLOOD BANKS FOUGHT RACIAL DISCRIMINATION

Something else that happened at Tuskegee was the Annual Clinic. Held every April by the Tuskegee Institute, it was a high point in the calendar for African American physicians from across the US, combining a medical conference with a free clinic for black southerners. On 1 April 1950, four doctors were travelling there from Washington DC when their car came off the road. The driver, Charles R. Drew (1904–50), died from his injuries the same day, and a legend sprang up that his death had resulted from white doctors' refusal to give him a blood transfusion. The legend was all the more potent because Drew had pioneered the large-scale collection and storage of donated blood.

Hospital blood transfusion services existed, but most relied on the patient's relatives and friends to donate blood as and when it was needed. In 1937, Bernard Fantus (1874–1940) opened the first US 'blood bank' at Cook County Hospital, Chicago, for the storing of blood for emergency use. Keeping blood in a usable condition, however, posed a problem.

Drew did his doctoral research at Columbia University, culminating in a dissertation titled *Banked Blood: A Study in Blood Preservation* (1940) which addressed blood storage problems. Through an experimental blood bank at Columbia's Presbyterian Hospital, he showed that separating the plasma from the blood cells prolonged the useful life of donated blood. Plasma on its own treated shock and loss of fluids, irrespective of the recipient's blood group – plasma was the same for everyone. Soon after receiving his doctorate, Drew was appointed Medical Supervisor of the Blood Plasma for

Great Britain project, organising the collection, storage and transportation of plasma to allies injured in the Second World War.

After this, Drew became medical director of the American Red Cross's blood plasma collection pilot scheme. In the summer of 1941, he returned to his true vocation – leading the department of surgery at Howard University, Washington DC, where he trained young African American surgeons.

It was then that an outrageous irony occurred. The Red Cross rolled out the pilot project but excluded non-white donors; Drew would not have been allowed to give blood to the project established through his expertise. Public protest forced a partial backtrack and everyone was permitted to donate, provided the blood was labelled according to race.

Drew was outspoken about this policy, calling it an 'indefensible one from any point of view' and asserting that there was no scientific basis for segregation. In 1947, he also lobbied the American Medical Association to change its membership rules, which effectively excluded black physicians. They weren't banned from joining, but all members were required to be in their county medical society, and for black doctors living in the south, that just wasn't going to happen.

The legends surrounding Drew's death emerged from this context, where segregated hospitals did refuse patients on the grounds of race. Drew himself was taken to Alamance County Hospital's emergency room, where the staff did all they could to save him, but his injuries were too severe. As his biographer Spencie Love has established, however, the legend represented a 'generic truth' about the exclusion of black patients.

94. Smoking Was No Longer Good for You

By the end of the nineteenth century, cigarettes had replaced pipes as the convenient and sophisticated way to inhale smoke. At the same time, lung cancer began to appear with greater frequency than it had ever done in the past. Studies such as one by Franz Müller in 1939 attributed the increase in lung cancer to the increase in smoking, and while evidence was inconclusive, the idea that cigarettes were bad for you began to gain ground.

Between 1930 and the early 1950s, tobacco companies responded to these threats by turning to the figure everyone could trust – the family physician. Avuncular, smiling, bespectacled men in white coats began appearing in advertisements, proclaiming that their favourite brand wouldn't irritate the throat. Physicians appeared as hard-working heroes, ready to attend patients in the middle of the night thanks to an energising few puffs. The local doctor, portrayed as a smoker himself, surely must be far more trustworthy than faceless scientific studies that didn't take into account real patients' situations.

As well as targeting the public, tobacco companies went direct to doctors themselves. It wasn't until 1953 that the *Journal of the American Medical Association* began refusing tobacco advertising; from 1946 until then, its readers were regularly informed that 'More Doctors Smoke Camels Than Any Other Cigarette'. Doctors picked up free samples at medical conventions and were exhorted to recommend their spluttering patients to switch brands for a healthier smoke.

In 1950, however, no fewer than five studies were published showing a strong association between smoking and lung cancer. By interviewing lung cancer patients about their smoking habits, Ernst L. Wynder and Evarts A. Graham in the US, and Richard Doll and Austin Bradford Hill in the UK showed an unmistakable correlation. The results of these two largest studies were backed up by the others. Doll and Hill concluded that 'smoking is an important factor in the cause of carcinoma of the lung'.

Doctors faded out of tobacco advertising, but they were coming in useful on the other side of the debate. Doll and Hill started a vast epidemiological study in 1951, designed to track future mortality from lung cancer and other diseases in thousands of smokers and former smokers. They chose doctors, who would be easy to keep track of via the Medical Register over the years (appropriately enough, this idea came to Hill while he was on the golf course!) The study, which followed 34,439 male doctors, ran until 2001, going on to show smoking's link to more than fifty diseases.

By 1960 there was no scientific doubt that cigarette smoking caused lung cancer, but the tobacco industry maintained that the issue was just a matter of opinion. Smoking might have declined in Britain but the industry has been quick to tap into 'emerging markets' elsewhere. In 2015, according to the World Health Organisation, there were more than a billion smokers in the world, with five million deaths directly attributable to tobacco use annually and a further 600,000 deaths among non-smokers exposed to second-hand tobacco smoke.

95. ORGAN TRANSPLANTS EXTENDED PATIENTS' LIVES

What is success? For me, it's making it to the end of the day without catching my sleeve on a door handle; for others, it's transferring a vital organ from one person to another and saving their life.

In the practice of kidney transplantation, success appeared bit by bit. Emerich Ullmann, a Hungarian surgeon working in Vienna, transplanted a dog's kidney to its own neck in 1902. Meanwhile, Alexis Carrel in France was developing the vein-suturing techniques that would become standard in transplant surgery. Over the next twenty-five years many surgeons experimented, but tissue rejection precluded long-term survival in transplant recipients.

The first human-to-human kidney transplant took place in 1933. Ukrainian surgeon Yurii Voronoy used a cadaver kidney for a patient who had attempted suicide, but she died. An attempt that wasn't entirely successful but achieved the goal of keeping the patient alive occurred in 1945 at the Peter Bent Brigham Hospital in Boston. Ernest Landsteiner, Charles Hufnagel and David Hume moved a kidney from a deceased surgical patient to a woman with renal failure. The organ was rejected after a few days, but had bought her enough time for her own kidneys to regain function.

Tissue rejection had to be overcome if transplants were ever to be a reality. British zoologist Peter Medawar (1915–87) reported in 1943 that multiple grafts transplanted from the same source were rejected more robustly each time, suggesting that the body had built up an immunological response to the new tissue.

There were still no immunosuppressive drugs in 1954,

but that year there was a breakthrough. Joseph E. Murray (1919–2012), also of the Brigham Hospital, led a team transplanting a kidney from a living donor. The patient, Richard Herrick, had an identical twin, Ronald, and Murray's team gave detailed consideration to the ethical implications of offering the surgery. The opportunity to perform a transplant with genetically identical material was surely not to be missed, but did they have the right to ask the healthy twin to make such a sacrifice? Consultation with clergy and lawyers enabled them to approach the Herrick family with confidence, and Ronald agreed to the procedure.

The operation needed careful planning; the surgeons got the brothers fingerprinted by the police to ensure they were really identical, and did a skin graft to test whether Richard's immune system would reject the tissue from Ronald. At 8.15 a.m. on 23 December 1954, the operation began, with John Hartwell Harrison (1909–84) undertaking the weighty responsibility of removing the kidney from the healthy donor. All went according to plan, and Richard spent Christmas in the care of the recovery room nursing supervisor, Clare Burta. After his recovery, they married and had two children. Richard lived for another eight years.

Most people's lack of a handy identical twin meant there was still much work to be done. The development of the immunosuppressive drug azathioprine by George Hitchings and Gertrude Elion, combined with Peter Medawar's work on tissue typing, enabled successful kidney transplants from non-related donors. In the early 1980s, cyclosporine further improved survival rates and became the standard way of avoiding tissue rejection.

96. THE BUILDING BLOCKS OF LIFE REVEALED THE PAST, PRESENT AND FUTURE

A bout of typhoid in 1869 gave Friedrich Miescher a career change. Miescher (1844–95) was training as a doctor, but the illness left him with hearing impairment and he felt this would compromise his communication with patients. He turned to biochemistry instead, focusing on the nucleus of white blood cells.

Where to get lots of white blood cells? Miescher struck a deal with the local hospital so that he could have old dressings off patients' wounds. With hospital infections still prevalent at this time, the bandages were covered in beautiful, creamy, glistening pus. His experiments revealed an unexpected non-protein substance inside the leukocytes' nucleii. He named it nuclein; it would later become known as deoxyribonucleic acid, or DNA.

Understanding of heredity was a big question. How did characteristics pass from one generation to the next and how did both parents contribute? The Danish botanist Wilhelm Johannsen coined the term 'gene' in 1909 but it was not until 1944 that Oswald Avery, Colin MacLeod and Maclyn McCarty demonstrated experimentally that DNA was the stuff responsible. Nine years later, James Watson (born 1928) and Francis Crick (1916–2004) at Cambridge described the molecule's structure – it was a double helix, an elegant twisted ladder of two chains of nucleotides, which could separate and act as templates for the replication of genes. Their work used data produced by Maurice Wilkins (1916–2004) and Rosalind Franklin (1920–58) at King's College, London.

Franklin and her PhD student Raymond Gosling (1926–2015) employed X-ray diffraction techniques to examine the structure of DNA. It was one of these images

– the iconic 'Photo 51' – that was to become central to the debate about the researchers' roles in the discovery. In the simple cross-shaped shadows of Photo 51 was the whole story of life; of origins and survival; of continuity and change. When Franklin was about to leave King's for Birkbeck in 1953, Wilkins shared her data with Watson, and it was crucial to supporting his and Crick's theoretical model.

Watson's memoir, *The Double Helix* (1968), fuelled controversy about this event. His chauvinistic attitude towards Franklin and his admission that he'd acquired Photo 51 without her knowledge did much to identify her as a wronged victim who had been cheated out of the Nobel Prize shared by Watson, Crick and Wilkins in 1962. The sense of injustice has encouraged widespread recognition of her contribution, but also overshadows her later achievements in establishing the structure of viruses. Franklin's death from ovarian cancer at just thirty-seven meant she could not be nominated for the Nobel Prize, and it is impossible to know how the Nobel committee would have viewed her work had she still been alive.

Knowledge of the structure of DNA has opened up new possibilities for medicine, with the development of gene therapy for hereditary disease, the ability to test genetic susceptibility to certain conditions such as breast cancer, and breakthroughs in personalised drugs for individual cases.

DNA enhances our understanding of the past – how early humans populated the globe and how they adapted to the challenges of survival. When it enables the prediction of future disease, it also raises the ethical question of how much we want to know about our fate.

97. A Devastating New Virus Was Identified in 1983

In the UK in 1987, every household received a leaflet featuring the stark word 'AIDS' chiselled onto a tombstone. In Australia, a notorious commercial warned that it wasn't 'only gays and IV drug users' being affected by HIV. Everyone was at risk from the Grim Reaper, who played a macabre game of ten-pin bowling, with people as pins.

It was six years since the first cases of pneumocystis carinii pneumonia (PCP) and Kaposi's sarcoma had begun to affect young gay men in the US, seemingly due to an underlying syndrome. Meanwhile, Ugandan physicians were observing Kaposi's sarcoma in young women. By 1985, it was established that the diseases were the same, and that people in every inhabited continent were affected.

HIV – Human Immunodeficiency Virus – is thought to have originated in chimpanzees and transferred to a bushmeat hunter in Central Africa in the early twentieth century. Acquired Immune Deficiency Syndrome (AIDS) occurs in the last stages of the disease, when HIV has severely compromised the immune system.

When AIDS reached epidemic levels in 1981, no one knew what it was; in a response reminiscent of long-ago plagues, people saw the disease as something to do with 'others'. Its early association with gay men fuelled existing homophobia, even as they mobilised to tackle AIDS through initiatives such as the UK's Terrence Higgins Trust. Although it soon became apparent that people from all walks of life were at risk, stigma has followed the disease all over the world.

The virus was isolated in 1983 by Luc Montaigner

(born 1932) and Françoise Barré-Sinoussi (born 1947) in Paris, and confirmed as the cause of AIDS by Robert Gallo (born 1937) at the National Cancer Institute in Maryland in 1984. (Cue much squabbling about who did what first, and a Nobel Prize for the French scientists in 2008.)

Within just a few years of the virus' identification, the first drug therapy, AZT, became available, focused on repressing the multiplication of the virus. Although there is no cure for HIV, since 1996 highly active antiretroviral therapy (HAART) has been able to reduce the viral load to undetectable levels, provided it is taken for life.

The question about treatment for HIV is now not whether it works but whether people can access it. Stigma remains a global problem preventing people from getting the care they need. Social ostracism, homophobia, job loss, violence, accusations of 'illicit' behaviour, and even hostile attitudes from healthcare providers deter people from seeking help.

In 2014, UNAIDS launched an ambitious target for the year 2020. By then, it aims that 90 per cent of people living with HIV worldwide will know their diagnosis. 90 per cent of those people will have full access to antiretroviral therapy, and 90 per cent of those receiving therapy will have an undetectable level of the virus in their body. The next step will be to end the epidemic by 2030. Whether this can be achieved depends on the availability and fair cost of drugs, the responsibility of governments to facilitate healthcare, and the commitment of communities to tackling the stigma that prevents millions of people from accessing treatment.

98. THE LAST NATURALLY OCCURRING CASE OF SMALLPOX HAPPENED IN 1977 …

Traditionally, the history of medicine has focused a lot on 'firsts' – the first to discover this, the first to realise that. Sometimes, however, it's just as significant to be the last.

The World Health Organisation launched its smallpox eradication programme in 1966, using a coordinated system of vaccination, isolation and statistical surveillance. This required the contribution of millions of health workers of all nationalities, many of them volunteers, who organised local campaigns, communicated the project to the public and overcame dangerous conditions to reach isolated communities.

Ali Maow Maalin (1954–2013) contracted smallpox when he was working at a hospital in Merka, Somalia. As well as his main job as a cook, he also volunteered with the WHO's smallpox eradication programme. When smallpox broke out in a nomadic community, a health worker brought two children suspected to have the disease to Merka, en route to the nearby isolation facility; Maalin travelled with the party to navigate to the camp. During this short journey, he contracted the disease, and on 22 October 1977, consequent symptoms appeared. Doctors confirmed the disease on 26 October, having initially suspected that it was chicken pox. He recovered, and no more naturally occurring cases of smallpox have been reported anywhere in the world ever since.

At the end of 2015, the last two official stocks of smallpox virus still lay in wait in high-containment laboratories in Russia and the US. Governments remained vigilant about their potential use in biological warfare, and the World Health Assembly (the WHO's main decision-making section) continued to debate the issue of when to destroy them.

99. ... AND ITS SURVIVOR WORKED TO ERADICATE POLIO

The success of the smallpox campaign served as a model for ending another lethal virus. In 1988, the Global Polio Eradication Initiative set out to put an end to polio by the year 2000. The campaign had to postpone its goal, but got results: the Americas were certified polio-free in 1994, the Western Pacific region in 2000 and Europe in 2002.

In 1996, African heads of state signed the Yaoundé Declaration, committing to allocate resources to the urgent eradication of polio. At the same time, Nelson Mandela launched the 'Kick Polio Out of Africa' campaign, calling on the continent's footballers to raise awareness of the disease and its prevention.

Ali Maow Maalin, the last person to have had naturally occurring smallpox, used his influence too. During a polio outbreak in 2004, he became the district polio officer for Merka, Somalia, organising vaccination clinics and using his story to convince people of the importance of vaccination. Speaking to the *Boston Globe* in 2006, Maalin said 'I want to be able to see the last person with polio. That's why I'm doing this.'

Although Somalia became polio-free in 2007, a new outbreak struck in 2013 and Maalin joined the response again, organising a vaccination campaign at Merka. While engaged in this work, he contracted malaria and died. He did not see the last person with polio, but his vision of a world without the disease was within reach. The Global Polio Eradication Initiative now aims to accomplish its goal in 2018, thanks to millions of volunteer health workers like Maalin.

100. No Action Today Means No Cure Tomorrow

Lilly Evans, my great-great aunt, was twelve when she came down with an ear infection in the summer of 1913. It was the kind of ailment that's usually just an inconvenience, but when it got worse the treatment options were limited. After nine months of chronic suppuration from her middle-ear, Lilly developed meningitis and died.

Streptococcus pneumoniae, the bacterium most likely to have killed her, proved susceptible to penicillin and, had she lived a few decades later, her life could probably have been saved. Yet a century after Lilly's death, antibiotic resistance threatens to make simple infections deadly once again.

Resistance is a natural phenomenon. Mutations allow bacteria to survive the onslaught of drug therapy; these surviving bacteria then reproduce, passing on the trait of resistance to subsequent generations and becoming a 'superbug' that shrugs off attempts to kill it. As well as *S. pneumoniae*, other resistant pathogens have been identified – among them, *E. coli* and Methycillin-resistant Staphylococcus Aureus (MRSA), a particular risk for hospital patients.

This situation is caused by the misuse of antibiotic drugs. Inappropriate prescribing, where healthcare practitioners lack up-to-date guidelines, is one part of the problem. In many regions, antibiotics are available over the counter in pharmacies, allowing people to see them as a quick fix for every ailment. The antibiotics used in agriculture to prevent costly animal disease and promote growth also contribute to the development of resistant strains. As the World Health Organisation's Director-General, Margaret Chan, warned in 2011: 'No action today means no cure tomorrow.'

The WHO reported in 2014 that even in countries running public information campaigns, awareness remained low, with many people still believing that antibiotics are effective against viruses such as the common cold. While you might see a poster warning against this at your GP's surgery and think 'Well, duh! Everyone knows that!' it's a sobering thought that in a 2013 European Commission survey, 49 per cent of the 27,680 respondents answered 'true' to the statement 'Antibiotics kill viruses'.

Resistance is a global problem, but economic and social inequality mean that those in under-resourced countries and areas of conflict suffer disproportionately. The WHO calls for consistent regulation of antimicrobial drugs, worldwide monitoring of resistance, a focus on infection control and awareness-raising among health professionals and the public. Their 2014 report warned that without concerted efforts on a global scale: 'A post-antibiotic era – in which common infections and minor injuries can kill – far from being an apocalyptic fantasy, is instead a very real possibility for the twenty-first century.'

This is part of the history of medicine and we're in it. Our 'now' features an astounding range of advanced treatments and once-impossible cures ... alongside health scams, emergent diseases and potential global health crises. For Lilly, the experience of blinding pain in 1913 was 'now'. Plague victims' view of the doctor's beaked mask was their 'now'; Ötzi's lonely death on a Tyrolean mountain was his 'now'. Through studying the history of medicine, we can attempt to understand the experiences and outlooks of our fellow humans in other times and places and appreciate that, while the circumstances of life change, the human condition remains the same.